Why Am I So Wacky?

How every woman can
eliminate the symptoms
of PMS, Perimenopause
and Menopause
naturally and safely.

by
Lorrie Medford, C.N.

LDN Publishing
P.O. Box 54007
Tulsa, Oklahoma 74155

WHY AM I SO WACKY?
How every woman can eliminate the symptoms of PMS, Perimenopause and Menopause naturally and safely.
ISBN #0-9676419-4-2
Copyright © 2004 Lorrie Medford, C.N.
LDN Publishing
P. O. Box 54007
Tulsa, OK 74155

Library of Congress Cataloging-in-Publishing Data
Medford, Lorrie, 1949
    Why Am I So Wacky?
    Lorrie Medford, C.N.
    International Standard Book Number: 0-9676419-4-2
    1. Hormone therapy 2. Menopause 3. Women's Health I.Title

NOTE: This book is not intended to take the place of medical advice. Readers are advised to consult their doctor or other qualified healthcare professional regarding treatment of their medical conditions.

Printed in the United States of America

10 9 8 7 6 5 4 3 2 1 First U. S. Edition

(For ordering information, refer to the back page of this book.)

The names of my clients have been changed. Any similarity to a real person is purely coincidental.

Contents

Foreword

Don't you find that just the mention of hormones, can make you crazy? It's hard to know which end is up when it comes to understanding our hormones. And I'm not just talking about menopause. More than ever before women of all ages are plagued with hormonal problems which include PMS, painful periods, irregular periods, fibroids, ovarian cysts, polycystic ovaries, fibrocystic breasts, endometriosis infertility, mood swings, low libido, depression, anxiety, lack of energy, insomnia, hot flashes, night sweats, weight gain, and bone loss. It's really difficult to enjoy life and feel good about yourself, when your hormones are raging out of control.

My own hormonal conundrum many years ago—anxiety attacks, night sweats, depression, low libido, lack of energy and weight gain—had me in a real fix. What began as a desperate need to find a solution to the symptoms which were causing havoc in my life led me to the most empowering information for regaining my hormonal balance and sanity. Not only did I find natural answers that resolved ALL of my symptoms but I also became a dedicated and passionate women's health crusader.

I learned that relying on drugs to deal with hormonal issues is a dangerous path. The U.S. government in December 2002 listed all steroidal estrogens found in HRT and the Pill as known human carcinogens. The findings from major medical studies have all concluded that the use of HRT is a major medical mistake. It makes absolutely no sense to prescribe carcinogenic hormonal drugs to women.

So what are we to do? The most important course of action is to get the right information and to commit to getting healthy!

Thank goodness for women like Lorrie Medford. Her many years as a Certified Nutritionist, researcher and author of numerous health books, have provided her with the experience and the knowledge to help us unravel the mysteries of our hormones. Her latest book, *Why Am I So Wacky?* clearly and concisely reveals the path back to hormonal balance. Not only does she lift the veil of confusion and misunderstanding that surrounds the causes of hormonal imbalance but, most importantly, Lorrie provides dozens of safe, effective and natural solutions

Women deserve hormonal balance at every stage of their lives. In *Why Am I So Wacky?*, Lorrie has written a great roadmap to help guide us there!

Sherrill Sellman
Author of *Hormone Heresy*
Tulsa, Oklahoma

Acknowledgements

I am most grateful to the thousands of female clients who have allowed me to help them walk through their hormonal journeys. Your testimonies are appreciated and they will certainly encourage other women to handle their hormonal symptoms naturally and safely.

Special thanks to my sisters, Jackie Johnson and Rabia Fournier who were both involved at various stages in the production of this book. I love you both and thank you for your prayers and encouragement! Thanks also to Lindsay Roberts and Wendy Tatro for taking time out of your busy schedules to read my manuscript and for your encouraging words and feedback.

Also, special thanks go to Dr. Donna Smith, a practicing Certified Clinical Nutritionist, for her wonderful comments, suggestions and edit. I really appreciate all of the time you have taken out of your busy schedule to read my manuscript, Donna. You are talented both as a nutritionist and editor.

I'm grateful for Dr. John Lee (author of *What Your Doctor May Not Tell You About Menopause, What Your Doctor May Not Tell You About Premenopause,* and *What Your Doctor May Not Tell You About Breast Cancer*). I'm so saddened by his death this past year. Dr. Lee was a pioneer in the field of nutrition and hormone balance, and his books will continue to educate women about natural solutions to hormone imbalances. Thousands of women's lives have been helped tremendously because of his work.

Very special thanks to hormone expert and internationally-known author, Sherrill Sellman. Sherrill, you are such a passionate researcher, writer, and advocate for women's health. Thanks so much for writing my foreword, and for your heartfelt concern for the health of women everywhere.

I'm always grateful to my own staff, Anne Spears and Carolyn Clark who manage to juggle client orders and appointments, while supporting the production of my books. Thank you both so much for all of your hard work and continual encouragement to write this book. Your gifts and friendship are so appreciated.

Many thanks to Lori Oller, for your edit. Your talent, focus and compassion are so appreciated.

I'm so aware that all of our gifts, talents and desires are given to us from God. So finally, I thank God with all of my heart. Every morning as my staff and I pray, we are grateful to have jobs where we can impact people's lives with encouragement, knowledge and good nutrition.

About the Author

Author and motivational speaker, Lorrie Medford has a B.A. in Communications and is a licensed Certified Nutritionist from The American Health Science University. She also holds certification as a personal trainer from ISSA (International Sports Science Association). She serves on the Board of Directors for the Society of Certified Nutritionists, and is a member of the Oklahoma Speaker's Association. Lorrie also serves on the Advisory Board for Standard Process, Inc.

In addition to writing this book, she has also written *Why Can't I Stay Motivated?*, *Why Can't I Lose Weight?*, *Why Can't I Lose Weight Cookbook*, *Why Do I Need Whole-Food Supplements?*, *Why Do I Feel So Lousy?*, *Why Am I So Grumpy, Dopey and Sleepy?* and *Why Eat Like Jesus Ate?*

A health researcher and journalist, Lorrie has studied nutrition, whole-foods cooking, herbs, health, fitness, and motivation for more than 20 years. Lorrie taught her weight-loss class at a local junior college and through her own business for more than 10 years, and has taught natural foods cooking classes in Spokane, Washington and Tulsa, Oklahoma for more than 5 years.

She shares her knowledge in her seminars, and through her thriving nutritional consultation practice, *Life Design Nutrition* in Tulsa, Oklahoma.

Lorrie has a rich history of community involvement teaching nutrition and is a sought-after speaker for civic groups, churches, hospitals, and wellness organizations.

She is uniquely qualified to write about health and fitness. Lorrie knows what it's like to be a *cranky calorie counter* obsessed with foods, dieting, and striving to be thin. After struggling with her weight for many years, Lorrie lost more than 35 pounds and has kept it off for more than nineteen years. She also manages to be hormonally balanced, in spite of her busy schedule!

Are You Confused?

Being a female health consumer is getting crazier by the minute. One day you hear on the morning news that estrogen protects you from deadly diseases such as osteoporosis and heart disease. The next day, you read an article about a study that reports that estrogen **causes** several types of cancer and is even linked to heart disease! All of this happens, of course, the same week you receive your first piece of correspondence from AARP!

Your neighbor takes some kind of "natural" hormones, but your doctor warns you against them. Never mind that he's never had a cycle in his life, and his wife is just as wacky as you! Totally confused, you wonder who to believe.

Sure, women have always had to deal with shifting hormonal levels, but today, so many things are different.
- Women are starting their cycles earlier.
- Women have more pain and other symptoms.
- Women are given more drugs for pain, acne and heavy blood flow.
- Their diets and lifestyles don't support proper hormone balance.

After I changed my diet more than 20 years ago, I stopped having PMS. And at 54, I haven't had any negative menopausal symptoms. I feel left out. I've never had to throw off the covers at night, and I don't have any excuses for my irritable behavior! Sometimes I'm tempted to eat chocolate fudge for a month just so I can experience a hot flash! If it weren't for all of my clients, I would miss out on all the fun! I have learned so much about hormonal mood swings and anxiety from working with women, that I could write another book in my "Why Can't I?" series entitled *Why Can't I Be Nice to My Family?*

While there are many books written on hormones, I wanted to write a book that simply dealt with the most frequently-asked questions that women ask me every day in my office. This book gives practical issues of diet, nutrition and lifestyle, based on experiences with my clients. For example, helping a woman manage her blood-sugar levels through diet goes a long way towards hormone balance.

In the past ten years, I've helped more than 6,000 women balance their hormones, including:

1. Prepare their bodies so they could get pregnant, after being unable to conceive for a year or more, and carry their healthy babies to full term.
2. Regain their cycles after skipping them for months.
3. Eliminate PMS and handle menopausal symptoms naturally.
4. Lose weight following some hormonal imbalance.

Where Do You Need Help?

Every woman has to deal with hormonal balance in her life, whether throughout her monthly cycle, or in menopause. Nearly every woman approaches me with the same simple questions:

- What about testing for hormones?
- Do I need hormone replacement? If I do, what kind is the safest and most effective, and how long do I need to take it?
- What about taking the Pill, calcium, Fosamax, and Tamoxifen?
- How can I get my husband to do the dishes? (Oh sorry, that's another book!)

In this book, I'll give you answers to these questions and nutritional solutions so you can get healthy and "balance" your hormones naturally without any risk.

Part One: Why Are Women So Wacky?

Part One is about hormone imbalances and the history of hormone replacement. We'll answer questions such as: Does HRT work? Is it safe? How did it begin? Do I need it?

Part Two: Beyond Standard Treatments for PMS, Menopause & Osteoporosis

Part Two looks at the standard treatments for female problems. You'll discover the real causes for PMS, hot flashes and being just plain wacky. I'll also answer questions such as whether or not synthetic hormones protect us from disease, and I will alert you to some of the dangers and side effects of drug therapies for menopause, PMS and osteoporosis.

Part Three: Natural Solutions for Hormone Imbalances

More than 25 million women are going through menopause, and for many of them, the symptoms can be unexpected, uncomfortable and unbearable. In Part Three of this book, I'll address frequently-asked questions and give you natural solutions to problems such as these:

- Fatigue
- Low sex drive
- Depression, mood swings
- Aches and pains
- Bloating and gas
- Hot flashes

- Weight gain
- Migraines and headaches
- Insomnia
- Lack of concentration
- Poor memory
- Hair loss

Part Three also looks at the vital connection between a woman's health and her hormone balance. You'll see why it's so important to eat well enough to keep your adrenal glands and liver healthy.

Part Four: Eating for Hormone Health

Part Four is about getting the right lifestyle for hormonal balance. We'll discuss exercise, good foods for hormone balance, and recommended supplements. I'll also recap the recommended nutritional supplements mentioned in this book.

Feel free to read this book all the way through or jump around. Okay, ready to get started? Let's begin with some simple tests.

PART ONE

Why Are Women So Wacky?

Chapter One

Are You Wacky?

Are you wacky for a week, once a month, every month? Do your mood swings include screaming at the top of your lungs when someone cuts you off in traffic? Or, do your hot flashes come so frequently that you have been able to lower your heating bill? What about crying because—well, anything will do! If any of this sounds like you at times—or all the time, then this book is for you!

There was a time when mothers passed down their dietary advice to help their daughters through menopause safely, but things changed in the late 1990s. People moved from the country to the city. Doctors replaced moms, and medical drugs replaced natural herbs.

Our mothers did the best they could. It's not like they could go down to Barnes & Noble and pick up a book entitled *Hot Flash Management for Dummies* or *The Idiot's Guide to Female Hysteria*. No, they weren't encouraged to discuss "The Change." So many of our female problems were either "mysterious ways of the female body" or "just in our heads."

Often, we heard our mothers say, "Welcome your cycle as a sign that you have become a woman." Did she forget to mention the migraine headaches, back pain and bloating? Try to convince the thousands of women who experience great hormonal shifts, weight gain, and mood swings that she should be glad she's a woman!

Where could women go for answers? (Male doctors don't understand what it's like to be a woman. And forget about asking your husband. You are lucky if your husband will stop and get you Mydol much less sanitary napkins. In fact, think of all the things that men miss out on—especially gynecological exams, mammograms and yeast infections. It's all more than any man wants to know or talk about!)

Women haven't been taught much about their bodies. Sure, we know that we have cycles every month—no one had to tell us about that! And we know that our ovaries make eggs that are able to be fertilized every month, and if there is no fertilization, we have another cycle next month. (For some this is great, for those trying to get pregnant, it's not!) But what about the other problems? Like pain before and during the cycle, skin break outs, and chocolate cravings?

Since the majority of the clients I've seen in the last 6-10 years are female, I've been involved in finding solutions to these common hormonal imbalances. There are ways to find the nutritional deficiencies, and yes, eliminate unwanted symptoms once and for all.

Let's start with a few basics. I've written three short symptom tests to determine possible hormone imbalances. (I'll discuss other ways to test hormones and their solutions in this book.)

Symptom Test One

1. Do you experience bloating and water retention?
2. Do you have breast tenderness or fibrocystic breasts?
3. Do you experience mood swings or irritability?
4. Do you experience anxiety and/or depression?
5. Do you have lower-back pain?
6. Do you experience cramps?
7. Do you experience fatigue?
8. Do you get headaches?
9. Do you have an increased desire for sweets?

10. Do you have acne or other skin eruptions?

11. Do you experience nausea or shakiness or dizziness?

12. Do you experience forgetfulness, confusion or decreased concentration?

While there are several reasons for many of these symptoms, if you have 1 or 2 of these symptoms, you are probably experiencing premenstrual syndrome, commonly known as PMS.

Symptom Test Two

1. Do you experience hot flashes or night sweats?
2. Do you have vaginal dryness?
3. Do you experience mood swings or irritability?
4. Do you experience anxiety and/or depression?
5. Do you experience irregular periods?
6. Do you experience unusual flow (too heavy or too light)?
7. Do you experience a decrease in libido (sex drive)?
8. Do you experience breast tenderness?
9. Do you experience bladder infections?
10. Do you experience insomnia?
11. Do you experience heart palpitations?
12. Do you experience urinary incontinence?

If you experience 2-3 of these symptoms, you are probably experiencing menopause.

If you have more of these symptoms than the PMS test, but you are not old enough to be considered in menopause, then you are in "premenopause," the 10-15 years prior to menopause. Premenopause is a term coined by hormone expert and author, Dr. John Lee. It generally refers to women who enter menopause in their late thirties and early forties, but it could even effect women earlier.

Perimenopause is the medical term that refers to the two or three years around the onset of menopause.

Symptom Test Three

1. Do you experience hot flashes or night sweats?
2. Do you have problems with your teeth?
3. Do you have any lower back pain?
4. Do you have joint pain?
5. Do you have leg cramps at night?
6. Do you have insomnia?
7. Do you have loss of height?
8. Do you have fair skin or freckles?
9. Do you have transparent skin?
10. Do you have arthritis?
11. Do you experience urinary incontinence?

If you experience 2 or 3 of these symptoms, you are one of those people who may be at higher risk for or have the beginnings of osteoporosis.

Unfortunately, experiencing any symptoms listed above is the "American way!" In case you wondered if you were the only one—no, you aren't! Unfortunately, it's unusual if you **don't** experience most of them.

In this book, I'll show you why these symptoms are far too common, and how easy they are to reverse, especially with the right diet and lifestyle. Unfortunately, most women don't get the nutrition they need from food, and many don't have the time to prepare meals properly. In my practice, most of my clients have asked me for nutritional supplements as well which are extremely beneficial in helping women alleviate symptoms as they make changes in their diets.

Ready? Let's start with looking at the history of hormone balance and how we got where we are today.

Chapter Two

What Is Hormone Balance?

We hear so much these days about hormone imbalance. People have made it sound so complicated. I simply tell my female clients, "If you suddenly notice you have an uncontrollable urge to surf the TV channels with the remote control in one hand and a lite beer in the other, then something's out of whack!"

Seriously, hormone balance is important, but I hope by the end of this book you'll also see that it's easy! You don't have to give up control of your body to others. The majority of my female clients are far more in tune with their cycles and know their bodies better than anyone. Women can experience menopause and monthly cycles as God intended—without symptoms.

The two major hormones that a woman produces are estrogen and progesterone. During the first half of her cycle, estrogen increases as her body gets ready for possible conception. This includes making the blood uterine lining for the baby's nourishment. In the second half of her cycle, estrogen levels decrease and progesterone levels increase. If conception occurs, progesterone levels increase even higher. She produces about 350 to 400 mg. of progesterone daily, which is required to maintain the pregnancy. If no pregnancy occurs, progesterone levels drop, the lining is shed, and the cycle starts all over again every month, until she reaches menopause.

In a perfect world, our bodies make the right amount of hormones. Our cycles come and go with no major symptoms of pain, headaches or depression. However, we don't live in a perfect world! There are numerous lifestyle conditions that cause women to become "out of balance." Let's look more closely at estrogen and progesterone.

Your Body Makes Estrogen

Estrogen is the major female reproductive hormone during the first two weeks of the menstrual cycle. Estrogen is the general name for several hormones that are naturally produced in the body: Estriol, estrone, and estradiol. Other hormones involved are pregnenolone, DHEA, testosterone, FSH and LH. In this book, we'll focus on these two major hormones, estrogen and progesterone.

Your Body Makes Progesterone

Progesterone is the major female reproductive hormone during the latter two weeks of the menstrual cycle. It's necessary for the growth and fertilization of the ovum and fetus.

Progesterone is a precursor hormone. That means it helps your body make estrogen, testosterone and all of the other important adrenal hormones. Since progesterone is so important, a deficiency of progesterone can cause problems including: Infertility, miscarriage, endometriosis, low thyroid, and fatigue. It's a pretty important hormone!

Natural progesterone, or the kind your body produces, is a health-promoting hormone. It can protect your body against fibrocystic breasts; it assists the normal functioning of your thyroid, and it's also a natural antidepressant. As you'll see later, it helps to maintain a normal sex drive and helps keep your blood-sugar level normal. One of the best benefits of natural progesterone is that it protects your bones against osteoporosis.

So What's Wrong With Me?

There are many ways a woman's hormones get out of balance, but by far the most common imbalance is an incorrect relationship between progesterone and estrogen levels.

We can have somewhat lower levels of estrogen near menopause, but our levels of progesterone are, relative to estrogen, dramatically lower. This creates a condition where we have more estrogen and less progesterone. This imbalance is called "estrogen dominance" a term that was coined by the late Dr. John Lee in his breakthrough book on hormone balance, *What Your Doctor May Not Tell You About Menopause.* Estrogen dominance means a decrease in progesterone levels to almost zero, with a decrease in estrogen only to about 50%. Dr. Lee felt that there are very few Western women truly deficient in estrogen. Most become deficient in progesterone.

So when your levels of estrogen are higher than your levels of progesterone, you are estrogen dominant. What are the symptoms of estrogen dominance? Nearly every negative symptom of PMS, premenopause, perimenopause, and menopause!

When estrogen becomes the dominant hormone in a woman's body and progesterone is deficient, then estrogen becomes too **toxic** to the body. Instead of causing good health, this imbalance causes symptoms of hormonal imbalance that can lead to disease. While this isn't yet named as a medical condition, I'm sure it wouldn't be called "EDD" for Estrogen Dominance Delight!

Let's look at the symptoms of this imbalance, who is estrogen dominant, and how we become estrogen dominant.

Let's begin with some common symptoms.

What Are the Symptoms of Estrogen Dominance?

What are the symptoms related to estrogen excess? Here's a list from hormone expert Sherrill Sellman's book, *Hormone Heresy:*[1]

* Aging
* Allergies
* Autoimmune disorders
* Breast tenderness
* Candida
* Chronic fatigue
* Decreased sex drive
* Depression
* Dry skin
* Endometriosis
* Endometrial cancer
* Excessive blood clotting
* Fibromyalgia
* Fibroids
* Fluid retention
* Gallbladder disease
* Hair loss
* Heavy periods
* Irregular cycles

* High risk of stroke
* High blood pressure
* Hirsutism (hair growth on face)
* Hypoglycemia (low blood sugar)
* Infertility
* Miscarriages
* Post natal depression
* Memory problems
* Migraines
* Osteoporosis
* Ovarian cysts
* PMS
* Skin problems
* Thyroid problems
* Uterine cancer
* Uterine fibroids
* Vaginal Dryness
* Weight gain (hips and thighs)

What Women Are Estrogen Dominant?

A woman's cycle should flow like clockwork—except in America—the land of "caffeine highs" and "sugar lows."

As women, we have several opportunities to become estrogen dominant—from the time we begin to have cycles as teens until menopause in our forties and fifties.

Why Are We Estrogen Dominant?

In my research, I've discovered four major reasons why women are estrogen dominant. Here they are:

1. ERT, HRT or Birth Control Pills.

Women who are taking synthetic estrogen replacement therapy (ERT or HRT) or Birth Control Pills become estrogen dominant due to estrogen excess. You may be wondering, if you are low in estrogen, how can you also be estrogen dominant? This can be confusing! But you can have low estrogen levels, and still be estrogen dominant, if your progesterone levels are lower than your estrogen levels.

2. Poor diet and lifestyle.

When women eat processed, fast foods, they don't get the proper nutrition required for hormone balance. No ladies, sausage biscuits and a coke are not a balanced meal!

Diet strongly influences women's hormones. And the very substances that she should eliminate are often the ones she craves! Substances, such as caffeine, coffee, soft drinks, black tea, chocolate, sugar, carbonated beverages, alcohol, hydrogenated oils, fried foods, vegetable oils, and preservatives all contribute to estrogen dominance. Our high-fat, high-sugar and processed diet leads to estrogen levels in women twice as high as women in third world countries.

In the 1900s, people ate one pound of sugar per person annually; today it's 200 pounds per person annually. Excess sugar is causing an epidemic of estrogen dominant women.

The American diet which contains processed foods and nutritionally-deficient foods provides insufficient nutrition to produce proper hormonal balance. And if you were raised on dairy products (who hasn't been in America?), then you have been bombarded with synthetic estrogens from hormones given to the animals. Now when you think about the average American woman's diet, it's easy to imagine that she could become estrogen dominant.

Too tired to work out? Additionally, a sedentary lifestyle is another cause for high levels of estrogen. Regular exercise has been clinically shown to lower high estrogen levels.

3. Taking certain medications.

Long-term over-the-counter and prescribed drug use over burdens and stresses the liver. A poorly functioning liver can also cause high estrogen levels because your liver helps to eliminate toxic hormones. We'll look more at the liver in Chapter 8.

4. Exposure to environmental estrogens.

There's another twist in this scenario. Plastics and petroleum-based products contain what is known as "xenohormones" or "xenoestrogens." (No, it's not Xena the Warrior Princess' hormone cream!) These are also referred to as "fake" estrogens.

Xenohormones describe chemicals that are foreign to our body and which block normal hormonal function. Xenoestrogens refer to a xenohormone that is estrogen-like, or acts like estrogen. Both can be found in some soaps, pesticides, and perfumes made from petro-chemicals.

The problem with xenoestrogens is that the molecule is so close in structure to the estrogen molecule, that your body interprets it as estrogen. So every time you have contact with these products, or eat foods with estrogen, your levels of estrogen rise! This then is another reason that women become estrogen dominant—the major reason for female hormone imbalance. Uh-oh!

Here is a short list of other xenoestrogen containing substances:

Xenoestrogen Containing Substances

· Synthetic hormone replacement	· Car exhaust
· Herbicides and pesticides	· Industrial cleaners
· Fingernail polish and remover	· Dry-cleaning fluids
· Alcohol	· Plastic wrap/containers
· Phthalates	· Plastic cookware

24

In case you were wondering, phthalates are compounds added to plastics to make them more flexible. They are found in the cling wraps used to wrap foods like cheeses and meats. Or they are in that "new car smell" used in various car parts. Plasticizers are used in: cosmetics, synthetic leathers, adhesives, caulking, insecticides, repellants, perfumes and so on.

Disorders Resulting From Xenoestrogen Exposure

According to Dr. Janet Lang, a practicing chiropractor who teaches classes on female hormone balance to doctors, these are the disorders related to xenohormone exposure:[2]

1. Increase in reproductive-site cancers in women and men (breast, uterine, ovarian, prostate, testicular).
2. Decreased fertility in both sexes.
3. Decreased sperm count in males.
4. Low testosterone levels and abnormally small penis size.
5. Increased PMS problems in women.
6. Estrogen dominance epidemic.

Between our fast food diets, junk food, stress, and exposure to chemicals, it's not hard to understand why so many women suffer with the pain and discomfort of hormone imbalance.

What Can I Do?

What can you do to minimize your exposure to xenohormones? Obviously, eliminating as many of these factors as possible is important for good health. Dr. Lang recommends the following.

   • Avoid all synthetic and horse hormones (see the next chapter.)

- Eat organic meat and dairy.
- Avoid the fat of non-organic meat and dairy.
- Decrease or stop all conventional pesticides and garden chemicals.
- Wear protective gloves and clothing when in contact with cleaning solutions.
- Buy cosmetics without xenohormones.
- Avoid synthetic-fiber carpets and fake woods.
- Ventilate properly when in contact with these materials.

(For people who would like to study this in more detail, you can contact Dr. Janet Lang at www.drjlang.com. for her seminars and tapes.)

There are a number of companies today that provide personal and household products that are free of xenohormones and chemicals. Check with your health food store or co-op.

Most American women have been estrogen dominant for quite some time. Yet, you might know that the most common medical hormone therapy is to give women more estrogen!

After reading this chapter, you might wonder then, how did the synthetic hormone replacement therapy begin? What type of clinical evidence was it based on? And finally, does it really work?

Let's move to the next chapter about the history of medical hormone replacement therapy and the impact it's had on American women.

Chapter Three

Who Decided How Women Handle Hormones?

Let's start this chapter with a somewhat possible scenario of a menopausal woman's appointment with a medical doctor.

She walks in and says, "Dr., I have been experiencing hot flashes," to which he quickly replies, "No problem. Take Premarin." Then he recommends Provera, a synthetic progestin which is recommended to offset the cancer-promoting effects of estrogen. She inquires about bone loss for which he recommends Fosamax, a drug for osteoporosis.

After being on hormones as the doctor prescribed, on her next appointment, she complains of high-blood pressure, for which he prescribes another medication. She's also just noticed lately that she tends to wake up in the middle of the night, so he gives her sleeping pills to help her sleep, such as Ambien.

On the next appointment, she tells him that the sleeping pills make her tired and depressed, so he gives her an antidepressant such as Prozac. She also finds that taking all of these medications now causes her heartburn, for which he prescribes Zantac or Tagament. Meanwhile, she's been on some type of thyroid hormone for years, but still she's overweight. And now she's beginning to experience hair loss. Hmmn. She's now on: Premarin, Provera, Fosamax, Ambien, Prozac, Zantac and Levoxyl. It's no wonder she's gaining weight! The combined side effects of all these medications could include weight gain!

What's wrong with this picture? As one client said, "All I wanted to know is why I have hot flashes, and I walked out with ten different medications!"

So many of my female clients come to their first appointment with me carrying the same combination of medications: Synthetic thyroid hormone, synthetic estrogen hormones, high-blood pressure medication and an antidepressant, asking, "How can I get off these?"

As I listen daily to these common female complaints, I wondered how did female hormone imbalances ever become medical conditions which require so many medications?

When Did Doctors Get Involved?

Did you know that until the 1940s, there were no synthetic hormone replacement pills? The idea of using synthetic estrogen as a hormone replacement began in 1966 when a gynecologist named Robert Wilson wrote about estrogen as though it were a type of magic pill that would keep women "feminine forever," which was the title of his book. None of the studies were definitive. Ten years later, more than half of American women were using estrogen, and doctors have been prescribing female hormone therapy ever since.

Dr. John Lee introduced the idea that **menopausal symptoms are a progesterone deficiency, not an estrogen deficiency.** He believed that menopause as a disease was largely fabricated by physicians and the pharmaceutical industry.[3]

Who really decided how women handle hormones? My guess is that since it was called "men-o-pause," men just decided they were the ones who had all the answers! (Does this mean that men go through "women-o-pause?" Even if men do experience some type of "Change," all they need to deal with it is a brand new corvette!)

Women Became Big Business

Women's health issues are huge business, to the tune of $15 billion a year! Pharmaceutical companies spend three billion a year to get women to take drugs. Author Sherrill Sellman says that drug companies target young girls with the Pill for acne,

PMS, and birth control. Peri and menopausal women are targeted for estrogen or estrogen/progestin combinations. She believes that all are expensive and dangerous.

In the last chapter, I said that a woman's body makes estrogen. Pharmaceutical companies also make estrogen. The most commonly sold synthetic estrogen is Premarin which means pregnant mare's urine because it is derived from estrogen found in horses' urine. In 1966, more than 22 million prescriptions were written for Premarin, grossing about $370 million. Premarin has been one of the top 10 prescription drugs sold in the U.S. since 1970, and more than 30 million women fill prescriptions yearly. Today, Premarin is still the most widely prescribed drug and it grosses about $900 million dollars a year.

Drug manufacturers dwarf the entire vitamin supplement industry which grosses about 6 billion dollars a year. A single drug can gross sales between 5-10 billion dollars a year.

According to Sherrill Sellman, between 750,000 to a million hysterectomies are performed each year. Three fourths of these are women under 49. Removing the ovaries forces her into premature, unnatural menopause, which then requires treatment.

The cost from these procedures is billions. When you want your dog to stop producing litters you castrate it. Surgically removing a woman's ovaries and/or uterus is female castration and is big money. The hysterectomy industry is worth 4 billion.[4]

Hysterectomies outnumber almost all surgeries in the U.S.!

Hysterectomies then promote big business for pharmaceutical companies because they sell all the hormone drug therapies that your doctors prescribe. For example, pharmaceutical companies make synthetic progesterones, called progestins. In the late 1800s a law was passed that medications could be patented only if they were **not** natural substances. Drug companies are not interested in natural substances; they want patents on drugs because that makes more money.

29

More About Money

Dr. Lee said that even fibroid growths have become a "money-making" disease. He explained that giving synthetic estrogen to a woman **before** menopause (for example, the Birth Control Pill) will cause fibroids to grow. Giving estrogen (hormone replacement therapy or HRT) to a woman **after** menopause will cause fibroids to continue to grow. Rather than change their diet or use appropriate supplements, the medical community recommends taking out the woman's uterus.

In an interview with Clinical Nutritionist Dr. Donna Smith, she said this would be like a doctor recommending that a man have his leg amputated because he complained of joint pain!

Here's a short list of potential problems after having a uterus removed: Fibrocystic breasts, weight gain, water retention, hypertension, blood clots, gallbladder disease, and the risk of breast or other hormone-dependent cancers. Every disease you could develop from this estrogen dominance condition means more money for your doctor and pharmaceutical companies. According to Dr. Lee, if you do something as simple as supplement with natural progesterone, you may never need to see your doctor in the first place![5]

With all of the surgeries, hormone replacement therapy and follow-up visits, the sad part is that thousands of women today are still dying of breast cancer, heart disease and osteoporosis. Yet no one is looking for the **cause** of these problems.

Does Synthetic Estrogen Work?

Estrogen is necessary for bone and heart health. And lower levels of estrogen can be responsible for hot flashes, irritability and many other discomforts. But the major medical solution for menopause for more than 30 years has been **synthetic** estrogen replacement therapy (ERT), instead of plant-based estrogens that do not have the dangerous side effects that ERT does. Common forms of synthetic estrogen are: Premarin, Estraderm,

Menorest, Esclim, Climara, FemPatch, Alora, Vivelle-Dot, Estinyl, Ogen, Ortho-Est, Estratab, Menest, and Cenestin.

Does ERT prevent menopausal symptoms? Nutritionist Shari Lieberman, in her book, *Get off the Menopause Roller Coaster* says that estrogen "does work some of the time, for some of the problems. It **may** help with osteoporosis, vaginal atrophy and thinning and hot flashes. It **does not help** with cardiovascular symptoms, fatigue, memory loss, irritability, loss of libido or difficulty with concentration."[6]

Hmmn, does this mean it's a little helpful? That's like me telling my client, "Take this vitamin. It **might** help you a little, but I hope it doesn't hurt you!" You wouldn't buy that. But daily, thousands of women around the country are encouraged to take hormones that help a little, but at a great price.

I've seen thousands of women, and more than half were on some type of hormone replacement therapy, yet they still experienced numerous negative symptoms. If this was the correct answer for menopause, why wasn't this "condition" totally cured or at the very least helped? Why hasn't the death rate from heart disease in women decreased?

Is HRT Dangerous?

Estrogen replacement therapy was never clinically proven to be safe and effective. In fact, during the late 1970s many reports were made public that linked estrogen replacement therapy to uterine cancer. So sales declined in the use of ERT and another form of hormone therapy was introduced, which added progestin (a synthetic progesterone) to the estrogen. So ERT changed to HRT, and doctors were taught **not** to prescribe estrogen alone. This new therapy is still called hormone replacement therapy (HRT). (I like to call HRT "Highly Risky Therapy," and ERT "Enduring a Ridiculous Therapy!")

However, now women take a synthetic progestin that causes all the same symptoms and disease that natural progesterone is known to prevent and protect!

Clearly, using estrogen alone still increases the risk for cancer. The pharmaceutical companies began to add synthetic progestin to protect women from the risk of cancers. However, with the use of two synthetic hormones, now there is **double** the risk of breast cancer.

According to Dr. Lang, here is the problem with synthetic hormones. Hormones fit into a cell receptor like a key fits in a door. Synthetic hormones aren't an exact fit. Like using the wrong key in a lock, this "jams" the cell receptor and changes the action. This is known as a side effect and it can be deadly.[7]

Synthetic estrogen is many times stronger than any woman's body would manufacture. It's also associated with a great risk of heart disease and several forms of cancer. Other negative side effects of synthetic estrogen are fibrocystic breast disease, and endometriosis. Synthetic estrogen depresses the thyroid, causing weight gain, (That alone would keep me from taking it!) yet it continues to be one of the top-selling drugs!

Provera is a synthetic progesterone. In his book, Dr. Lee gave the side effects of Provera, the most common synthetic progesterone used in treating menopause. He listed five specific warnings, eight contraindications (or conditions that would prohibit use of the drug); six precautions, ten adverse reactions (including breast tenderness, acne, hirsutism, and weight changes), and five conditions that are observed when Provera is taken along with synthetic estrogens (including headaches and hair loss). You can read more about this in the Physicians' Desk Reference (PDR).[8]

Common forms of synthetic progesterone, called progestins, are: Provera, Amen, Cycrin, Alygestin, Micronor, Norlutin, Norlutate.

I interviewed Cynthia Drasler, a former pharmaceutical sales representative/sales trainer for chemotherapy:

> When I started selling chemotherapy in 1962, I was told that the breast cancer rate for women in this country was 1 in 14. When I quit the industry in 1990, the breast cancer rate for women in this country was 1 in 9. Now, I've been told that it is

approaching 1 in 7. **Obviously, something is very wrong with the way women are being treated in this country.**

By 1975, numerous reports linked uterine cancer with estrogen medications, and sales of estrogen medicines dropped. However, shortly after that, massive marketing campaigns touted the "benefits" of synthetic estrogens and doctors again told their patients that they **needed** estrogen for protection from heart disease and osteoporosis regardless of their risk for these diseases. Questions never asked were: Did they ever do a bone density test? Were they even at risk for either disease?

The average woman doesn't have the time or medical background to question this original research. This was information that you had to discover on your own.

According to Dr. Earl Mindell, author of *Prescription Alternatives,* taking Premarin for more than a year increases the risk of cancer of the endometrium by as much as 14%. Women on HRT (Premarin and Provera) may increase their risk of breast cancer by as much as 30%. For every 1,000 women using one of these drugs, 30 will develop breast cancer from the HRT itself.[9]

The pharmaceutical manufacturers themselves give a combined total of more than 120 potential risks and problems associated with HRT.[10]

Let's now look at some clinical studies on these hormones.

Some Larger Clinical Trials

Recently there have been two major studies published showing that conventional hormone replacement therapy (HRT or ERT) does more harm than good. You may have read about these studies in major newspapers or heard about them on television news shows.

The first study published was from the huge Women's Health Initiative and included 16,000 women. This study which was supposed to be for 8 years, had to be stopped three years early when results showed that women using Premarin and Provera or PremPro had a 29 percent higher risk of breast cancer, a 26 percent higher risk of heart disease, and a 41 percent higher risk of stroke.

The second study from the Breast Cancer Detection Demonstration Project showed that estrogen-only hormone replacement (ERT) increases the overall risk of ovarian cancer by more than 3-fold. According to Dr. John Lee, giving **only** estrogen to women without a uterus should never have become a medical protocol; yet doctors still do this.

The most disturbing part of the increasing risk for disease for Dr. Lee is that it was created due to the carelessness of conventional medical practice which dictated—without good supporting evidence of safety and efficacy—that **any woman over 50** complaining about anything remotely related to menopause be put on ERT. Their hormones weren't measured to determine what they needed or how much. Rather, they were subjected to a "one-dose-fits-all" mindset that created overdoses of estrogen for millions of women. Furthermore, the efficacy of progesterone in hormone replacement had been totally ignored in favor of the patentable (and therefore more profitable) synthetic counterparts known as progestins.[11]

Major Cover Story

"The Truth About Hormones" was the cover story for the July 22, 2002 issue of *Time Magazine*. In it, Christina Gorman and Alice Park asked many questions which should have been asked 30 years earlier regarding the benefits and risks of HRT. They site the Women's Health Initiative as definitively showing for the first time that the hormones in question—estrogen and progestin—**are not** the age-defying wonder drugs everyone thought they were, and to the contrary, proved that taking these hormones increased a woman's risk for disease. The principal message is this: Taking (synthetic) estrogen and progestin for years in the hope of preventing a heart attack or stroke can no longer be considered a valid medical strategy.[12]

After reading the results of these studies, you could wonder when making money became more important than healing women. I've wondered how synthetic estrogen and progesterone could even stay on the market for all these years! Didn't they care enough to study the effects of hormone replacement therapy before now? So often I've heard female clients tell me their doctor said, "Oh, it won't hurt you!" On what clinical basis did they make such statements?

Why Doesn't Your Doctor Know?

Doctors still don't understand natural hormone balance. Dr. Johnathan Wright, M.D. gives us a peek into the life of the average doctor. He reports that most doctors are completely in the dark about the use of natural hormones. (As if you didn't know!) They aren't taught about natural hormones in any medical school. Drug companies are the other major source of information for nearly all "conventional" physicians. Almost all doctors only see studies of the benefits and risks of Premarin, Provera, and other patentable hormones. These are studies which the pharmaceutical industry has conducted itself or underwritten.[13]

Who Should Help You?

First, realize that you can become your own hormonal expert, especially as you begin to take responsibility for your health and improve your diet and lifestyle.

Second, the type of "natural" health professional you want to assist you in health improvement are Naturopathic Doctors (N.D.), Certified Nutritionists (C.N.), Certified Clinical Nutritionists (C.C.N.), and any doctor (D.C., M.D., D.D., D.O., D.D.S., Ph.D.) or pharmacist who completed post-graduate studies in Clinical Nutrition.

So let's move on to Part 2 and look further at PMS, menopause and osteoporosis.

PART TWO

Beyond Standard Treatments for PMS, Menopause & Osteoporosis

Chapter Four

PMS

Once a month the symptoms begin. Headaches, bloating, and "Please, just get me chocolate!" We call it PMS, or pre-menstrual syndrome. Many husbands call it, "Punish My Spouse!" Or as television teacher Joyce Meyer says, "Pretty Mean Sister!" (I prefer to call it "Pretty Moody and Sweaty!") It usually occurs 7 to 10 days before menstruation and stops when the period starts. Up to ninety percent of American women experience some type of PMS.

It's not bad enough that women struggle through their cycle, but for many they struggle two weeks ahead of their cycle and two weeks after their cycle as well! In a good month, some women may have about twenty minutes without any symptoms! For all the water retention, it's a good thing that bell bottoms are now back in style!

Did you ever notice your cycle usually happens at the least opportune time; like when you are on the highway, fifty miles from a rest station, on an airplane without any tampons (in the middle seat!), or the only time you borrow your best friend's new silk dress?

If you don't have physical symptoms, then you recognize it by the need to send hubby out at any hour—day or night—to buy M&Ms. (Yeah, like that's going to help you!)

Since there is no laboratory test for PMS, women have had to become their own experts in figuring out what's going on. They will go to great lengths; even attending social gatherings with a thermometer under their arm! Never mind waiting for their doctor to finally figure out a healthy solution. They've got hot flashes or crying spells now! Best of all, women know how to talk to each other and compare notes! Here's Sally taking to Mary under the hair dryer at the salon: "Your hot flashes are gone? What are you taking and where did you get it?"

What's Normal?

A normal cycle begins when a female reaches 12 or 13, comes regularly every 28-30 days and lasts about 3-5 days with little if any symptoms of pain, cramps, headaches or unusual bleeding. However, few American women experience "normal" cycles!

In my weight-loss book, I mentioned that in China, girls reach menstruation between ages 15 to 19, which is more natural. Unfortunately, due to estrogen dominance from the foods they are eating, I've even heard of young girls in America starting their cycle between ages 8 to 10! This isn't normal because the cycle brings with it ovulation and the opportunity for pregnancy. These young girls are not emotionally or physically ready for sex and/or pregnancy.

Another part of abnormal cycles is the varying negative symptoms. About 14 million women experience PMS with over 150 documented symptoms associated with it, mostly in the two weeks before menstruation. These symptoms are magnified after taking the Birth Control Pill, after pregnancy and before menopause.

All PMS symptoms reflect a highly toxic condition! Here are common symptoms of PMS:

PMS-A: Anxiety, including insomnia and irritability

PMS-H: Hyper-hydration, including water retention problems, bloating, and breast tenderness

PMS-C: Cravings, including cravings for sweets and increased appetite

PMS-D: Depression, including forgetfulness and confusion

PMS-P: Back pain and headaches[14]

Nearly every symptom listed is a symptom of various vitamin and mineral deficiencies and stress. Here are some examples. (See Chapters 7-9 for further help.)

Phobias and Panic Attacks: Anxiety is related to both vitamin B and C complex deficiency combined with various other deficiencies including magnesium. They can also be caused by low-blood sugar and mineral deficiencies.

Bloating can be related to circulation problems involving digestion, gallbladder problems, vitamins B, C and E complex deficiencies, B6, magnesium and essential fat deficiencies. Bloating may also be caused by mineral imbalances, such as a low potassium to sodium ratio.

Breast tenderness can be helped with Vitamin E, flaxseeds, Evening Primrose Oil or Black Current Seed Oil.

Cravings for chocolate can indicate magnesium deficiency. Cravings for carbohydrates or sugars can indicate zinc or chromium deficiencies.

Depression is linked to folic acid deficiency, Omega-3 fatty acid and B complex deficiency and is also related to both estrogen and progesterone deficiency or zinc to copper imbalance. (More about this in Chapter 7.)

Back pain and headaches are related to a prostaglandin imbalance. Helpful support includes progesterone, Evening Primrose Oil (expensive) or Black Current Seed Oil (less expensive), and Dong Quai. Headaches may be caused by copper toxicity, low-blood sugar, toxic metals, chronic infections, allergies or mineral deficiencies. Also, rubbing progesterone cream on her abdomen can relieve cramps.

There are a myriad of other problems with menstrual cycles. Let's look at a few of these more closely.

Excessive Bleeding (Menorrhagia)

Excessive bleeding with clotting and cramping can be due to a fibroid tumor, where the blood is bright red instead of the normal dark red. Inflammation of the uterus may cause bleeding, but the blood is dark. Fibroids can also cause cramps.

In addition to balancing your hormones, your natural health professional may suggest iron, progesterone supplementation, or help from herbs such as Crampbark for pain, and Capsulla for heavy bleeding.

Painful Menstruation (Dysmenorrhea)

Uterine cramping is common the first few days of the cycle, and can last several days. It's usually caused by inflammation or irritation of the ovaries, uterine fibroids and/or liver stress.

Common treatment includes eliminating estrogen dominance as outlined in this book, supporting the liver (See Chapter 8), and balancing blood-sugar levels (See Chapter 9).

No Cycle (Amenorrhea)

A common reason for lack of a cycle is that the woman is not eating enough good, essential fats. Cholesterol is required for your body to produce hormones. (Yes, you can be too thin!)

Secondly, perhaps the woman is experiencing excessive amounts of stress or she is exercising excessively. Very irregular cycles are a common symptom of estrogen dominance as well. (See Chapters 7, 8 and 9 for additional help with these symptoms.)

More information is provided in Chapter 7 regarding PMS symptoms similar to the above-list such as mood swings, breast swelling, cramps, and fatigue.

Conventional medical treatments for all types of PMS include antidepressants, tranquilizers, diuretics, anxiety medications, and synthetic hormones such as the Birth Control Pill. However, I've learned from my female clients that most medical treatments have side effects that are worse than the original symptoms. Surprisingly, many doctors deny that PMS even exists. They consider these conditions as "in the woman's head." These doctors certainly don't seem to understand that imbalances in the nutritional biochemistry affecting a woman's hormones can cause physical and emotional problems. However, that's what I've seen day-in and day-out in my nutrition practice for the last 6 years.

What Really Causes PMS?

In an interview with Clinical Nutritionist Dr. Donna Smith, Ph.D., she stated the root causes for PMS:

> PMS is caused by stress, our typical American diet, drug therapy and toxicity which all cause various vitamin and mineral deficiencies. These contribute to organ and gland dysfunction including the liver, thyroid and adrenals. These dysfunctions then cause the hormone imbalances that produce PMS, and all female symptoms from puberty to menopause.

Let's look at the most significant hormone imbalances and organ/gland dysfunction that leads to female complaints.

1. Progesterone deficiency. Symptoms of PMS are similar to symptoms of estrogen dominance, so one of the most common causes of PMS is progesterone deficiency during the second phase of a woman's cycle.

Progesterone has been wrongly accused of being the hormone responsible for PMS because it's the one that's high right before menstruation. However, women with PMS have lower progesterone levels than normal at that time in their cycle when progesterone should be dominant.

There are a couple of popular ways to increase a woman's level of progesterone. One is to use the herb Chaste Tree and the second is to use a progesterone supplement. (See Chapter 8 for more information.)

2. A sluggish liver. Hormone balance depends on how fast and effectively the liver can remove estrogens. Many women have a sluggish liver; it's not a diseased liver, but a liver that's not able to effectively eliminate excess estrogen and toxins as it's designed to do. More importantly, most women should do an internal cleanse for their whole body, including the liver, colon and other organs of elimination.

What causes a sluggish liver? The same foods that I mentioned earlier that cause estrogen dominance: Alcohol, caffeine, sugar, refined carbohydrates and trans-fats. Too much fat, too much dairy, too much salt, sugar and processed foods contribute to an imbalance of hormones and liver stress. Fiber plays an important role: Lack of fiber can cause estrogen to be reabsorbed and recycled. (See Chapter 8.)

3. A sluggish thyroid. Hypothyroidism can cause symptoms of PMS, fatigue, headaches, loss of sex drive, and infertility.

4. Stress and adrenal problems can also cause severe anxiety symptoms related to PMS. (See Chapter 8.)

Dr. Janet Lang gives several theories about causes of PMS (If this is too technical, just know that eating better helps!):[15]

1. Abnormal response to normal hormone levels
    a. Cell membrane malfunction often because of trans-fats
    b. Imbalances or excesses of other hormones such as cortisol (an adrenal hormone)
2. Elevated prolactin levels
3. Xenohormone exposure in the uterus and/or as a growing, developing child
4. High refined carbohydrate diets, hypoglycemia and/or insulin resistance
5. Eicosanoid imbalance
6. Nutritional deficiencies, especially in magnesium, zinc, copper and B complex vitamins
7. Stress which effects steroid hormone balance
8. Candida infection
9. Altered brain chemistry

Premenstrual Dysphoric Disorder (PMDD)

Even our monthly cycles can be a means of big business for the pharmaceutical companies. In his book, *Women's*

Health Solutions, author Gary Null interviewed Sherrill Sellman about the history behind a "new" female disorder called Premenstrual Dysphoric Disorder (PMDD), that is treatable with a "new" drug called Sarafem. Sherrill says that first of all, the symptoms of PMDD are the same as PMS. **It is not a new disorder.**

She explains that when Eli Lily, the maker of Prozac, lost the patent on Prozac, he convinced the FDA to create this "new" condition for which their drug and only their drug can help. This of course, is so they can continue to keep Prozac on the market. However, it's the **same** drug, but only packaged differently in a pink and purple pill.[16]

You might wonder what's wrong with taking something like Prozac? Clearly, as I've said earlier, PMS and PMDD are **not** Prozac deficiencies. But more importantly, Sherrill warns that Prozac can be highly toxic to the liver, it can cause mood swings and brain damage, suicidal thinking, and puts women at risk for breast cancer. Sherrill says, **"Women need to wake up to the fact that again they are being sold a bill of goods, that this is not the solution, and that the motive behind it is purely profit."**[17]

What About the Pill?

Recently, a young female client, who was struggling to lose weight told me she was taking the Birth Control Pill. Sometimes doctors prescribe the Pill for female problems with acne, or heavy periods (for which I have many natural nutritional solutions). When I asked her why she started taking it, she said that she just didn't want to be bothered with cycles anymore!

God made every woman to have a normal cycle. This means every month, from age 13 to 50, she could conceive. According to fertility experts, there are only 3 or 4 days a month when she is actually fertile. Having a cycle, however, is a way for a woman to detox every month, and some people have theorized that this could be why women live longer than men.

I can understand why a woman would not want to experience a horribly painful cycle. However, suppressing the body's natural processes of having hormonal cycles by taking drugs is not the answer because it puts her at high risk for cancers of the female glands later in her life.

How the Pill Works

The Birth Control Pill or Patch is designed to suppress the menstrual cycle. The theory is that without a cycle a woman would not experience cramps, PMS, endometriosis, ovarian cysts or hormonal acne.

But in order to suppress or override such a natural process, hormones must be **higher than normal levels,** either from synthetic estrogen and synthetic progesterone (progestin) or as an implant or injection made with progestins such as Depo-Provera or Norplant. This process increases estrogen dominance which in turn causes serious hormone imbalances with high risks.

Author Sherrill Sellman says that stopping a woman's natural reproductive cycle can sometimes permanently damage her ovaries and even lead to infertility.[18]

Even though as early as 1932, it was known that estrogen and progestins could cause cancer of the breast, womb, ovaries and pituitary glands in animal experiments, the Pill was believed to be a good solution to the overpopulation crisis. Although it was known early on that the Pill caused blood clots, it wasn't until the mid 1970s that the death toll for young women taking the Pill got public attention.

Sellman calls the Pill "dangerous and a potentially life-threatening steroid drug that causes grave harm to women."

She believes that women need to be educated about the dangerous hormones they are putting in their bodies.[19]

Side Effects of the Pill

Women so casually take the Pill, it's clear that they have no idea about the serious side effects. Often they are taking it while either not experiencing immediate effects, or ignoring the subtle (allergies) or not so subtle (weight gain) side effects.

Here are two lists, both major and minor side effects from Sherrill Sellman's *Hormone Heresy* book.[20]

Major Side Effects of the Pill

- Disturbance in blood-sugar metabolism
- Increased risk of stroke
- Increased risk of blood clots
- Increased risk of gall bladder disease
- Increased risk of hardening of the arteries and high blood pressure
- Liver tumors
- Possible link with cancer of the endometrium, cervix, ovaries, liver and lungs
- Increased risk of ectopic pregnancy
- Three to six-fold increase in the risk of heart attacks
- Osteoporosis

Minor Side Effects of the Pill

• Allergies	• Breakthrough bleeding
• Decreased immune function	• Disturbances in liver function
• Eye disorders	• Facial and body hair growth
• Fluid retention	• Fungal infections
• Hair loss	• Hay fever, asthma, skin rashes
• Loss of libido	• Lumpy breasts
• Migraines	• Nausea
• Emotional disorders	• Secretions from the breast
• Skin discoloration	• Suicide
• Weight gain	• Urinary-tract infections
• Vaginal discharges	• Varicose veins

Recently a client came in wearing a once-a-week Birth Control Patch, saying it helped keep birth control and PMS "off her mind." I had to enlarge the accompanying package insert 210% on my printer before I could read the very, very fine print. The adverse reactions included: ...breast symptoms, headache, application site reaction, nausea, upper respiratory infection, menstrual cramps, and abdominal pain. Serious adverse reactions included a risk of blood clots, myocardial infarction, gallbladder disease, and benign liver tumors.

Surprisingly, included in the last list of side effects (which said, "neither confirmed nor refuted") was pre-menstrual syndrome. This is one of the symptoms the Patch was supposed to treat! After explaining the serious side effects of taking the Birth Control Patch, my client told me, "I would have to be 'out of my mind' to keep using this Patch!"

Vitamin Deficiencies

As if all of these drug-related side effects weren't enough, additionally, the Pill interferes with how vitamins are absorbed. Sherrill Sellman reports that the Pill causes major nutritional deficiencies including vitamin A, B1, B2, B6, Folic/B12, C, E, K, and minerals magnesium, zinc and copper.[21]

The combined effect of these vitamin and mineral deficiencies can include fatigue, weight gain, and serious problems with fertility and birth defects as in the case of the B vitamins and especially folic acid.

While the medical solution is to "medicate" the symptoms of PMS, a better approach is to understand the cause of these symptoms and find that solution. You'll learn more about how to handle common symptoms in Chapter 7.

However, changing your diet, and handling stress will go so very far in handling most of these PMS symptoms. See Chapters 8 and 9.

Let's move on to the next stage of a woman's life, often accompanied by recommendations for more synthetic hormones and/or surgery.

Chapter Five

Perimenopause and Menopause

What happened to the good old days when we could eat anything and never gain weight, and get by on 3 hours of sleep a night? Today, we consider that a nap!

Perhaps you're too young for menopause, but just when you thought you might be finished with PMS symptoms, they linger on and on. You're probably thinking, If I'm not in menopause, can't I at least be finished with PMS? We have enough to worry about! For example, I'm still trying to figure out why, when I put on lipstick, it ends up on my teeth!

Dr. John Lee coined the PMS type-symptoms in older women, ten to twenty years before menopause "premenopause." Think of it as a dress rehearsal for the real thing! Symptoms include: Bloating, weight gain, headaches, depression, irritability, memory loss, cold hands and feet, fibroids, tender breasts, weight gain, problems with conception, fatigue and irregular cycles that can be light or heavy. **He believed it's not a natural part of life, but is caused by our culture, lifestyles and environment.**

If you have regular cycles with these symptoms, it's PMS. However, when your cycles become extremely irregular, you are probably in premenopause. Premenopause generally refers to women not old enough to experience menopause, yet suffering from many symptoms of menopause and PMS.

What About Perimenopause?

As if it's not confusing enough, there is yet another phase of a woman's life: Perimenopause. The word "peri" means around, so perimenopause refers to the 2-3 years just before menopause, during which a woman's cycle changes to irregular cycles and even lack of cycles. It's common for cycles to be irregular for one or two years up to menopause. However, even though women aren't in menopause, they may still have symptoms including hot flashes, insomnia, lower sex drive, and depression or anxiety. Since the average age of menopause is 51, most American women start perimenopause between ages 47-48.

When Is Menopause?

Skipping twelve monthly menstrual cycles in a row is what most people call menopause. It begins gradually over a fifteen-year period starting anywhere from ages 35 to 50. Your ovaries gradually decline in the production of estrogen and progesterone. Ask your mother when she experienced menopause, since heredity can be involved, but more commonly, diet and lifestyle are involved.

Menopause due to surgical removal of the ovaries occurs in 30% of U.S. women. Cigarette smoking has an effect on menopause, causing it to occur 1 to 2 years prematurely.[22]

Every woman, if she lives long enough will experience "The Change." Currently there are about 40 to 50 million women who are postmenopausal. Some dread it, but not as much as their husbands! (The good news is you can't get pregnant anymore; the bad news is you may have lost your libido and you can't find it!) There are benefits, though, such as no more cycles or cramps once a month, and no more sugar binges. Now you just get to grow a beard!

Symptoms of Menopause

In a healthy woman, there are no uncomfortable symptoms! I've learned through my practice in helping thousands of women that the healthier they have been throughout their lives, the easier menopause will be. That means they followed a good diet, exercised regularly and managed their stress. (Did you ever notice that "managing stress" really means they got their husbands to take the kids to soccer practice, do laundry, and clean the kitchen?)

However, it's more normal to experience symptoms, because of our high-stress and fast-paced lifestyles. Most American women experience any of the following:

- Hot flashes and night sweats
- Water retention
- Weight gain in the hips and thighs
- Decreased sex drive
- Bone loss
- Sleep problems
- Vaginal dryness
- Mood swings
- Headaches or migraines
- Thinning hair
- Fatigue
- Aches and pains
- Dry skin
- Lack of concentration
- Facial hair growth

But do we really have to go through all that? No! Surprisingly, most experts in the field of natural hormone therapy think not. Every day, hundreds of women are discovering that God did have a plan for them, and it was good! Just as your body naturally prepared you to be able to become pregnant, later, it prepares you to enter another natural stage of life. Or, as my twin sister, Jackie, says, "The egg factory is shutting down!"

I've been "menopausal" for a year and I don't have the symptoms that so many of my clients experience. It's not a dreaded time at all. (It's about time I felt good! I was overweight and a compulsive overeater for many years!)

As you might have guessed, the key to balancing hormones at any of these stages is a balanced diet, regular exercise and stress management. However, often women who come to me for help have been so "wacky" for such a long time, that they need additional nutritional therapies to help them with these symptoms as I teach them about following a healthier lifestyle. Therefore, it's important that women be nutritionally tested so they can take the right whole-food supplements to improve hormone balance whenever they experience any female symptoms.

We'll look at how to manage symptoms in Chapter 7; in this chapter I'll discuss the common medical treatments.

What Happens at Menopause?

The most obvious thing is that your cycle stops. Here's where you can save a lot of money on Tampons, Mydol and sanitary napkins! (But I'm wondering what to do with all these boxes of leftover tampons. I'm thinking of emailing Martha Stewart. Maybe she has great tips on making Christmas decorations with them!)

For years, doctors have believed that at menopause, estrogen drops, and for that reason estrogen has been routinely prescribed for estrogen deficiency.

Author Sherrill Sellman says that estrogen levels drop to only 40-60%, just low enough so that the egg follicles do not mature, so pregnancy is impossible. The ovaries do not shrivel up nor do they cease functioning. They continue to be productive endocrine glands. Only the outermost part of the ovary shrinks. The innermost part of the ovary, known as the inner stroma, actually becomes active at menopause.[23]

In the medical community, menopause isn't just a natural stage of a woman's life; it's a disease. And the prescription, as I mentioned earlier, is synthetic estrogen for the rest of your life. Yet, few women need estrogen after they clean up their diet and balance their hormones.

Menopause is not a "disease" that has to be treated. I have many clients who admit that they didn't want to be pressured into taking any hormone replacement therapy, and so they didn't—and they have had few, if any, menopausal symptoms.

What About Women in China?

If menopause were truly a disease, it would be a universal one. And looking at how other cultures pass through menopause without any symptoms shows us otherwise. In China, women have few, if any, symptoms of menopause. They don't even have a word for menopause in their Chinese language. Can you imagine that? Americans, however, had to create the word "menopause" just because of the negative affects of a fast-paced, junk food, drug-oriented lifestyle that has caused women to experience a variety of symptoms.

It's time to think about changing our lifestyles to support our health instead of tear it down.

What makes Chinese women different from American women? Their diet is generally a low-fat, high-fiber one. Their menopausal experience is driven by a good diet and healthy lifestyle. Studies show that if they move to the U.S. and follow our typical diet, they begin to experience the same symptoms as American women.

Does Estrogen Protect You From Disease?

The common medical solution for menopause has been estrogen therapy because estrogen has been touted as the "cure-all" for many symptoms of menopause, but particularly to protect a woman from heart disease, osteoporosis and Alzheimer's.

One of the problems with ERT or estrogen replacement therapy is that estrogen alone is dangerous, as I mentioned earlier in this book. Many conventional doctors now prescribe progestin, a synthetic progesterone, along with estrogen. Otherwise, the risk of endometrial cancer is too great. Doctors commonly prescribe Premarin, (horse urine) which increases her chances of breast or uterine cancer.

The obvious advantage of using "natural" plant estrogens is that they provide the same benefits of synthetic estrogens without the side effects, and protect women from breast and uterine cancer. See Chapter 7.

After menopause, the risk of serious heart disease including high-blood pressure, stroke and heart attacks appear to rise dramatically. Heart disease is the leading cause of death in postmenopausal women. So it is important to understand how to protect women from heart disease.

For years, it's been believed that synthetic estrogen protected a woman from heart disease. Hormone researcher and author Sherrill Sellman says that the overzealous prescribing of synthetic hormones to menopausal women to protect them against cardiovascular disease **is based on faulty data** and has caused a rise in heart attack and stroke incidence in these women.

Sellman reports that synthetic estrogen and progestins, the two key ingredients of oral contraceptives, have been responsible for strokes, blood clots and heart attacks in women taking the Pill.

Sellman also reports that synthetic progestins (Provera) co-administered with estrogen counteract any beneficial effects estrogen may have in preventing heart disease and stroke, and increases the risk of coronary vasospasms. Even the packet insert of the combined estrogen and progestin pill, Prempro, warns, "taking estrogen may increase the risk of blood clots. These clots can cause a stroke, heart attack or pulmonary embolism, any of which may cause death or serious long-term disability."[24]

One study commonly cited that said estrogen prevented heart disease was the Boston Nurses Questionnaire Study. Dr. Lee said the study was radically flawed and the statistics manipulated. Although there was ample evidence from numerous studies showing that the opposite is true—that estrogen is a significant factor in **creating** heart disease, these findings have been ignored. Dr. Lee said that the pharmaceutical advertisements neglected to mention that stroke deaths in the study were 50 percent higher among the estrogen users.[25]

Hormone author Dr. Susan Love's theory about this is simply that heart disease is heart disease. She says that it's more common in postmenopausal women because they are older than pre-menopausal women. It's like gray hair; you're more likely to have gray hair after menopause than before, but menopause doesn't cause gray hair.[26] (By the way, the primary cause of gray hair is mineral deficiencies.)

Real Risk Factors for Heart Disease

According to Dr. Love, the combined factors listed below are what put you at risk of a heart attack:[27]

• Family history can indicate whether you've inherited genes that make you more susceptible to the atherosclerotic process.

• Lipid Levels: Many factors influence the levels of LDL and HDL, including insulin, diet, exercise, obesity, age, and hormones.

• Homocysteine is thought to damage the inner lining of arteries. Studies show that the B vitamin supplements, especially folic acid, reduce homocysteine levels.

• Diabetes: Uncontrolled diabetes of either type have a treacherous effect on the small arteries throughout the body.

• Smoking at least triples the risk of coronary heart disease.

• Overweight: Obesity is a strong risk factor for coronary heart disease in women.

• High-blood pressure can lead to heart attacks by increasing the stress on the blood vessels.

• Blood clots make someone more prone to heart disease.

Most of these factors are involved with diet and lifestyle. Rather than using synthetic estrogen replacement therapy, let's look now at some healthy solutions for preventing heart disease. Though you can't change your family history, you can change your lipid levels.

For years, people have blamed all fats and saturated fats in general for heart disease. One of the main culprits linked to heart disease that is commonly overlooked is trans-fatty acids. Trans-fats as they are known, come mostly from hydrogenated vegetable oils. This is a process where a vegetable oil is made into a solid. This process, however, damages your arteries. In 1999, the FDA proposed a ruling to put trans-fats on food labels. However, to date, nothing has been done.

Eating "good" fats such as the kind found in cold-water fish and flaxseeds can lower cholesterol and protect your

WHY AM I SO WACKY?

heart. Additionally, high-levels of insulin have been implicated in high triglycerides and cholesterol. Eating a low-carbohydrate diet and taking the herb, Gymnema, has been extremely helpful for this. (See Chapter 9.) Other incredible nutrients for your heart include the following.

Recommended support for your heart:
- **Garlic and Ginkgo**
- **Magnesium/calcium**
- **Vitamin B, C and E complex**
- **Essential oils (Omega-3 fats)**
- **Hawthorne**
- **Regular exercise and stress management**

Estrogen and Your Brain

For 20 years, synthetic estrogen has been touted as the answer for Alzheimer's. The first study on estrogen and Alzheimer's included only 12 women, yet it was believed to be "the proof" that estrogen prevents Alzheimer's. The latest study showed that it was not effective in protecting women and that long-term estrogen therapy is dangerous to a woman's brain. It doubled the risk of dementia![28]

The best approach if you feel you may have a higher risk of Alzheimer's is to follow a nutritional preventive program.

Recommended support for preventing Alzheimer's:

- **Antioxidants can prevent cell damage in the brain. Vitamins A, C, E and the mineral selenium are great antioxidants as well as grapeseeds.**

- **Essential oils (Omega-3 fats).**

- **Circulatory support: Ginkgo and Vitamin E complex.**

- **Nerve support: B complex vitamins.**

- **Following a healthy, balanced diet is vital. Eliminate caffeine, sugar, fried foods and alcohol.**

Now let's move on to the next chapter on bone health and osteoporosis.

Chapter Six

Osteoporosis

Osteoporosis affects more than 25 million Americans, and it's no longer just our grandmothers who have it. Half of all women between the ages of 45 and 75 show beginning signs of osteoporosis; one in three will have full-blown osteoporosis; and by age 75, the number jumps to 9 in 10. However, osteoporosis is largely preventable and treatable.[29]

(As if women don't have enough to worry about with age spots, crow's feet and wrinkles. Of course the most common cause of wrinkles and aging appears to be raising children!)

Osteoporosis means porous bones, or brittle bones filled with small holes. Nutritionist Carl Germano author of *The Osteoporosis Solution,* defines osteoporosis as "A progressive disease in bone mass and density, causing skeletal weakness and brittle, fragile bones that are subject to breaking."[30]

The most vulnerable bones are the hip, wrist, shoulder, rib and spine which can make fractures more likely.

Is It a Disease or Risk Factor?

In the book, *Dr. Susan Love's Hormone Book,* the author questions the definition, asking, "Why not define low bone density as **a risk factor** for osteoporosis, rather than as osteoporosis?" Calling it a warning sign can eliminate needless fear. Once you are told you have a "disease," you look for treatment. Drug companies and doctors know this and Dr. Love calls this a driving force behind some new "diseases." Women who learn they have low bone density are more likely to be put on some type of hormone replacement therapy. However, they are rarely given information on what their bone density test means.[31]

Are You At Risk?

In *The Wisdom of Menopause,* Dr. Christiane Northrup lists each of these as affecting hormone balance that becomes a risk factor for osteoporosis:[32]

- Family history of osteoporosis
- Quite thin or tall
- Spending most of your time indoors
- Sedentary lifestyle or fitness fanatic
- Sluggish liver
- Clinically depressed
- Early menopause
- Taking anticonvulsant medication
- Below normal bone density tests
- Fair-skin and blue-eyes
- Smoking
- Amenorrhea (no periods)
- Drinking alcohol
- Drinking coffee
- Poor diet
- Taking steroid drugs
- Thyroid disorder

Hormones and Bones

To understand how we "get" osteoporosis, we have to understand how bones are formed.

Throughout your life, your body breaks down old bone tissue that's worn out (resorption) and replaces it with new bone tissue. The process of breaking down and rebuilding bone is called remodeling. From the moment you are born, to about age 35, your skeleton continues to grow until it reaches peak bone mass. From this age on, you begin to lose more bone than you build.

Hormone expert, Dr. John Lee explains that in osteoporosis, more bone is broken down (being resorbed) than is being made new. His groundbreaking book on progesterone, that I've mentioned throughout this book, *What Your Doctor May Not Tell You About Menopause,* shatters several myths about osteoporosis regarding calcium, estrogen and menopause.[33]

Shattering Common Myths

The first myth is that osteoporosis is a calcium deficiency disease. Lee found throughout many years in following his female clients, that while they took calcium supplements, it didn't prevent osteoporosis. Calcium was lost more than it was added, regardless of how much calcium a woman took. Clearly there were other factors involved.

The second myth is that osteoporosis is an estrogen deficiency. Dr. Lee called this, "A fabrication of the pharmaceutical industry with no scientific evidence to support it." He explained that osteoporosis begins long before estrogen levels fall and accelerates for a few years at menopause. Estrogen can slow bone loss, but it cannot build new bone.

The third myth is that osteoporosis is a disease of menopause. Lee discovered, through his clinical practice, that osteoporosis begins anywhere from five to 20 years prior to menopause, when estrogen levels are high![34]

What About Drugs?

Synthetic estrogen was considered "safe" for menopausal symptoms, yet for more than 30 years, it's been prescribed for women for osteoporosis with dangerous results.

Drugs, even when prescribed by physicians, are dangerous. Realize, too, that properly prescribed and over-the-counter drugs kill between 100,000 and 200,000 people in the U.S. a year.

Sherrill Sellman considers osteoporosis just another way for drug companies to make more money. "Women are told that the war on bone loss requires calcium supplements. Doctors also strongly recommend long-term use of estrogen to the postmenopausal woman, and additional help from drugs like Fosamax. Over the next 20 to 30 years armed with this powerful arsenal, a woman is told she will be able to walk tall and fracture free. Unfortunately, this is far from the truth."[35]

Osteoporosis has spawned a phenomenal growth in the drug industry. "The sale of just one estrogen drug, Premarin, grossed $945 million dollars in 1996. The U.S. Dairy industry is thriving with its annual 20 billion dollars in 1996.

And sale of calcium supplements spirals into the hundreds of millions of dollars."[36]

Sandra Coney, author of *The Menopause Industry* cites, "In the 1990s, the reorientation of osteoporosis as a woman's disease is complete. It is now mandatory to include osteoporosis as a major 'symptom' in any discussion of menopause. By convincing the public and the medical profession that osteoporosis is a crippling 'killing' disorder and estrogen the only cure, HRT has been imbued with a kind of saintliness."[37]

The switch from HRT as a treatment to HRT as a preventive therapy occurred without any discussion.

Dr. Jerilynn Prior, researcher and professor of endocrinology at the University of British Columbia has conducted research that seriously challenges estrogen's key role in preventing bone loss. Her research confirmed that estrogen's role in combating osteoporosis is only minor. As a result of her extensive research, she confirmed that it is not estrogen, but progesterone, which is the key bone-building hormone.[38]

What About Calcium?

The makers of calcium supplements also claimed that their products could prevent bone loss despite the fact that there is no absolute evidence that this is true. Sellman says, **"Scientific evidence shows unequivocally that, by themselves, calcium supplements just don't work."**[39]

The real key here is a synergistic balance of all bone-related vitamins and minerals, such as calcium with vitamins D, F and phosphorous, just to name a few.

According to Sherrill's *Hormone Heresy Supplement,* dairy products contribute to bone loss. Those countries that consume the highest amounts of dairy products also have the highest rates of osteoporosis; the non-dairy consuming countries have the lowest osteoporosis rates.[40]

Medical Treatment

There are several drugs being used to treat osteoporosis, and according to the author of *Prescription Alternatives,* Earl Mindell, none work very well, and all have unpleasant side effects. Fosamax (Alendronate) is the preferred treatment, the only non-hormonal drug approved by the FDA to treat osteoporosis. Medical doctors receive four-color advertisements stating that Fosamax is the newest and best thing for building bone. Studies of this drug were stopped after four to six years, the point at which the fracture rate for women taking similar drugs began to rise. Why? Because unfortunately, the old bone is structurally unsound, and after three to six years tends to increase the rate of hip fracture.[41]

According to Dr. Lee, Fosamax is a biphosphonate, a family of non-hormonal drugs which have been tested for over 20 years. Biphosphonates can dissolve human cells so they are found in tub cleansers to remove soap scum.[42] There are four biphosphonates currently in clinical use: alendronate (Fosamax), etidronate (Didronel), risedronate (Actonel) and pamidronate (Aredia). They stop bone resorption. They poison the osteoclast (cells responsible for removing damaged bone) so the old bone can't be removed, which makes bone denser—not necessarily stronger.

However, after five years, bones get weaker! Biphosphonates don't build new bone, so now the bone fractures can start. This has happened with all biphosphonates; all have been tried and abandoned. The 1988 Physicians Desk Reference (PDR) cautions against long-term use of this drug saying that bone formation is ultimately reduced!

You can't override the body's normal system of bone building (the removal **and** replacement of new bone) and expect perfect bones! (Except in the made-for-TV movies; anything is possible there!) More than that, there are many side effects.

For example, Fosamax can burn a hole through your esophagus and stomach; the manufacturers know this. That's why they have a warning on the label about "severe inflammatory reaction." They say in small print, to be sure not to lie down after taking it because it will burn a hole through your intestine.

Side effects of both Fosamax and Didronel include: Severe heartburn that can cause permanent damage to the esophagus, stress on the kidneys, impaired fertility, diarrhea, low calcium, vitamin D deficiency, magnesium deficiency, flatulence, rash, headache and muscular pain. Rats given high doses of these drugs developed thyroid and adrenal tumors.

Another medical treatment for osteoporosis is raloxifene (Evista). It's marketed as an alternative to women who can't take estrogen but want to prevent osteoporosis. According to the package insert, Evista can cause hot flashes and blood clots and is linked to a high risk of ovarian cancer.

The Most Important Factor

The most important factor in the beginning of osteoporosis is the lack of progesterone, which causes a decrease in new bone formation. In fact, Dr. Lee believed that there is no better treatment for osteoporosis than the progesterone supplementation.

Dr. Lee explained in his third book, *What Your Doctor May Not Tell You About Breast Cancer,* that estrogen inhibits the process by which old bone is removed to make room for new bone, or slows bone loss. Progesterone, on the other hand, **stimulates new bone formation** through special cells called osteoblasts.[43]

Adding progesterone will actively increase bone mass and density and can reverse osteoporosis. In his book, Dr. Lee cited a 72-year old woman who experienced a 29 percent increase in bone mineral density in less than three years of progesterone therapy.[44]

Bone-Density Testing

The American Osteoporosis Foundation recommends that women age 65 and older have bone-density tests every year. If you are under 65, and especially if you have any of the risk factors listed earlier, you should also have a bone-density test.

DEXA is an X-ray of your spine or hip that shows the loss of calcium. A cheaper test is a portable DEXA machine that measures the bone density in your heel. Other options for testing are ultrasound heel reading, saliva or urine test.

Preventing Osteoporosis

A healthy diet combined with progesterone therapy is your foundation! Eat lots of fresh fruits and vegetables, lean protein and few carbohydrates. Ditch the sugar, caffeine, soda and alcohol which cause calcium loss. High-calcium foods include yogurt, tofu, sardines, salmon and leafy greens.

Take calcium and other bone-related nutrients. But taking the wrong kind of calcium won't build bone if you are eating an acidic, fast-food, processed diet! Avoid calcium from ground-up rocks, as in calcium carbonate. (See my book, *Why Do I Need Whole-Food Supplements?*)

In order to absorb calcium, you'll need hydrochloric acid (HCl). People who take antacids and acid-stopping medications can't make enough HCl and put themselves at risk for osteoporosis.

Recommended help for preventing osteoporosis:
· **Hydrochloric acid**
· **Magnesium/calcium/manganese**
· **Vitamins D and K**
· **Essential oils (Omega-3 fats)**
· **Natural progesterone supplementation**
· **Support digestion and thyroid**
· **Regular aerobic and resistance exercise**

Let's go to handling the symptoms of hormone imbalance.

PART THREE

Natural Solutions for Hormone Imbalances

Chapter Seven

How To Handle Common Symptoms

As we women get older, have you noticed that our conversations often move from the latest fashions or hairstyles to more important things like what we take for our hot flashes, joint pain, and how to stay regular!

The economy may be downsizing, but we baby boomers see increase along the lines of double chins and expanding waists and hips! Wisdom comes with age, but does it make up for cellulite, falling hair and sagging body parts?

And the worse thing is that while going through all of these changes, we are continually reminded by a series of hot flashes throughout the day!

Hot Flashes

For those of you who are unfamiliar with them, most women report that it feels like your body slowly begins to heat up. Hot flashes can feel like a slightly warm feeling, or a stronger rush of heat overtaking you. They can happen in the daytime, or in the evening, as night sweats where many women often wake up drenched. It's even worse when you have them in the middle of a hot summer. At least in the winter, you could lower your heating bill!

As with other symptoms, the healthier you are before you reach menopause, the less you will experience hot flashes. Since stress is related, the better you handle stress, the less you will experience hot flashes. (So especially now is not the time to worry about the missing socks in the dryer!)

In working with thousands of clients over the past 12 years, I've discovered several reasons for hot flashes:

1. A decline in estrogen.
2. An imbalance of estrogen to progesterone (estrogen dominance).
3. Having a hysterectomy or partial hysterectomy.
4. Smoking.
5. Possibly having low-blood sugar conditions.
6. Being a thin woman with a lower percentage of body fat.
7. Following a toxic, junk food diet and stressful lifestyle.
8. Toxic bloodstream or colon.

Additionally, there are certain triggers that seem to be related to hot flashes. According to Dr. Linda Ojeda, author of *Menopause Without Medicine,* these are common triggers:[45]

• Hot weather, drinks, clothes	• Spicy foods
• Caffeine (coffee, tea, chocolate, colas)	• Exercise
• Vigorous lovemaking	• Alcohol
• Drugs of all kinds	• Large meals
• Meals eaten too quickly	• Stress

How can you eliminate them? Let's start with diet and lifestyle suggestions, and then add nutritional supplement suggestions.

Eating a healthy diet to maintain normal blood-sugar levels, while supporting the adrenal glands and liver is vital. Eliminating white sugar, white flour, and caffeine products is also important, as all of these substances upset normal blood-sugar levels. Have balanced meals of protein, carbohydrates and good fat, with plenty of vegetables and fruits. (See the recommendations listed in Chapter 9.)

Take care of your blood-sugar levels by eating regularly, every 2-3 hours. Keeping your blood sugar stable will help to control hot flashes. And drink plenty of water. You'll want to drink 1/2 your body weight in ounces of pure water every day. Just drinking more water has eliminated hot flashes for many of my clients.

Get a food diary and diligently write down everything you eat for a week or two to notice the relationship between your hot flashes and your diet. Often food triggers such as caffeine and sugar, clearly are connected to hot flashes.

Getting enough sleep, handling stress, and getting regular aerobic exercise can reduce hot flashes. The more exercise you do, combined with good diet, the less hot flashes you will experience. Exercise strengthens every part of your body, especially the adrenal and thyroid glands and is vital for everyone.

Helpful Supplements for Hot Flashes

· **Progesterone cream** alone is a wonderful help for many clients that I have counseled, especially if their hot flashes are really a symptom of estrogen dominance, not estrogen deficiency. Some Clinical Nutritionists also recommend sublingual (under-the-tongue) progesterone. Progesterone should be used with professional guidance from your natural health care professional. (More on progesterone in Chapter 8.)

· **Black Cohosh and Dong Quai** are two of the most thoroughly researched herbs for reducing the symptoms of menopause, including hot flashes, sleep problems, and depression. Sage, Panax Ginseng and Siberian Ginseng (Eluthero) are also good for hot flashes.

· **Black Cohosh** is also proven effective against hot flashes, anxiety, mood swings, low libido and vaginal dryness. Combined with a good diet and exercise, it works tremendously.

· **Red Clover** is one of the richest sources of phytoestrogens—plants which contain estrogen-like substances. It contains genistein and diadzen, as well as formononetin and biochanin, which are not found in soy.

· **Chaste Tree** or sublingual natural progesterone can also reduce hot flashes and other menopausal symptoms.

· **Foods high in phytoestrogens** are apples, carrots, celery, cherries, dates, garlic, peppers, oats, onions, pears, yams and soy. Many of my clients have reported less hot flashes just by eating one serving of tofu a day when estrogen deficient. (See the other side of soy on page 95.)

· **Ground flaxseeds** are also a great source of phytoestrogens and fiber. Fiber helps lower estrogen dominance. It binds to excess estrogens and helps eliminate them.

· **Additionally, a natural source of vitamin E** has been helpful for many of my clients. The best food sources are: wheat germ and wheat germ oil, whole grains, nuts and seeds, and olive oil.

Eat lots of broccoli and spinach for good food sources of boron and magnesium, both wonderful for calming the body.

Weaning off synthetic estrogen also can cause hot flashes; work with your natural healthcare professional. When women continue to have hot flashes in spite of the dietary changes and supplements, I recommend they follow a liver detoxification program. When the liver is sluggish it can't metabolize estrogen properly, so "excess" estrogen circulates, causing a rise in estrogen, or symptoms of estrogen dominance. (See *Why Can't I Lose Weight?*, and my book on cleansing, *Why Do I Feel So Lousy?*)

Food Cravings

Since hormone imbalances involve the liver, nearly every woman with a sluggish liver will experience PMS or menopausal cravings. Additionally, most women eat too many carbohydrates which sets them up for high insulin levels causing weight gain and even insulin resistance.

The first thing to do is balance blood-sugar levels by eating small amounts of protein for breakfast, lunch and dinner. Additionally, use the following:

- **Sugar cravings:** Chromium GTF, Zinc, or Gymnema
- **Chocolate cravings**: Magnesium
- **Salt cravings:** Use Celtic sea salt from a health food store

Skin Problems

Skin problems around the cycle can indicate progesterone deficiency. Check for possible allergies and digestive problems, since skin problems can indicate poor digestion and a sluggish liver and colon.

- **Digestive enzymes**
- **Natural progesterone supplementation**
- **Vitamin A complex**
- **Zinc**
- **Acidophilus supplement**
- **Liver/body detoxification**
- **Essential fats (Omega-3)**

Anxiety and Heart Palpitations

Anxiety is always linked to magnesium and/or progesterone deficiency and adrenal stress. Eating a good diet is important, as many of my clients have a history of excess caffeine and sugar for years which causes several mineral deficiencies and further stresses the heart, adrenal and thyroid glands. I encourage my clients to check with their doctor for heart problems, thyroid or adrenal issues.

- **Eliminate all stimulants (for example, coffee, tea, soda & sugar)**
- **Eat regular meals**
- **Magnesium helps to calm down the heart palpitations**
- **B and C complex, Valerian Root and adrenal support**

Depression and Mood Swings

Hormones influence emotions! An imbalance of estrogen in a woman and testosterone in a man can cause brain fog, the lack of the ability to concentrate and depression. Dr. John Lee confirms this link in his *July 2001 Medical Letter.* He writes that estrogen decreases thyroid function, based on an article in the *New England Journal of Medicine.*[46]

When Janice, a female client came to see me she was taking many drugs, including several antidepressants, and told me at the end of the appointment, that if I hadn't given her some answers, she was going to commit suicide that day! I put Janice on a trans-dermal progesterone cream before she left my office. Within three days, she sent me flowers, saying how much better she felt and that her crying had stopped. Within two weeks she was back to work, after struggling for the past year. She's still doing well with the nutritional changes and supplements I recommended.

There are links between nutritional deficiencies and depression. Unfortunately, most teenagers with PMS and depression live on junk foods and diet sodas or beverages loaded with caffeine. Just eliminating the stimulants, such as coffee and sugar can help eliminate depression. Not only do these foods and beverages cause B vitamin deficiencies, but in addition, teens rarely eat foods with the B vitamins. Early signs of B deficiency are characterized by depression. Serious B deficiency symptoms are: anxiety, hostility, emotional instability, craving for sweets, mental confusion, and irritability. You can get B's from eating eggs, nuts, seeds, nutritional yeast and meat. Additionally, getting enough good fat from cold water fish or flaxseeds helps with depression.

Depression is commonly due to estrogen dominance from low thyroid. Thyroid support includes the B complex, iodine, E complex, selenium and zinc.

Drugs such as Wellbutrin and Prozac are commonly used for depression. Side effects of Wellbutrin include: restlessness, agitation, dizziness, dry mouth, nausea, vomiting or constipation. Side effects of Prozac include rash, nausea, drowsiness, anxiety, dry mouth, and decreased libido. Drugs commonly used for panic disorders include Xanax and Zoloft. Side effects of both Xanax and Zoloft include drowsiness, dizziness, and headaches.

While these drugs are popular, realize that they are not getting to the cause of depression. Let's face it. If we all exercised regularly and ate right, we wouldn't need any drugs! The biggest problem I have with antidepressants is that most of the time they cause weight gain, which as you might have guessed, causes more depression! Besides, a good diet combined with natural substances is effective and without side effects.

St. John's Wort has been used for thousands of years, it is medically approved for the treatment of depression, anxiety and insomnia in Germany. Sales there outnumber all other antidepressants. If you decide you want to try St. John's Wort, do not take it while you are already taking an antidepressant.

Ginkgo and ginseng can help as well as acidophilus and a liver detoxification program. See your health professional for thyroid support. (I use Thytrophin by Standard Process which you can only buy through a licensed, health professional, not over-the-counter.)

Recommended supplements for depression:
- **Natural progesterone supplementation**
- **Vitamin B complex**
- **Folic acid/B12**
- **Essential oils**
- **Ginkgo/ginseng**
- **St. John's Wort**
- **Probiotics and liver detoxification**
- **Check thyroid and adrenal gland**
- **Regular exercise is helpful to treat and prevent depression**

Memory Loss

Isn't it sad, that as we age, our memory goes, but we sure can retain water! Never mind trying to remember names and phone numbers of our friends and family; some of us are so forgetful that we can even forget our own names!

Drugs and stimulants such as caffeine, tobacco and alcohol accelerate brain activity, but then later depresses its function. But the worse thing for memory? Sugar, sugar, sugar! Diets high in white sugar decrease blood sugar to the brain as well. (For more information on diet and exercise to prevent depression see Part 4.)

Scientific research shows that eating a type of fat called Omega-3 fatty acids, helps the brain to function better. It also helps with mood and memory. Omega-3 fats are found in cold-water fish (such as salmon and tuna) and flaxseeds. Women who eat Omega-3 fats while pregnant can decrease their chances of developing postpartum depression.

Recommended supplements for memory:
- **Essential oils (Omega-3)**
- **Vitamin B complex and Folic acid/B12**
- **Ginkgo to improve circulation and boost memory**
- **Ginseng for alertness, memory and concentration**
- **Probiotics and liver detoxification**
- **Regular exercise**

Fatigue

Just when we think we'll only be dealing with cellulite, wrinkles and aging, we have another issue: fatigue! Fatigue is rarely due to just one thing. Below is a list of possible energy robbers. This list may be overwhelming, but as you'll see, most are related to diet, nutrition and lifestyle. (For more information, see my book about fatigue, entitled *Why Am I So Grumpy, Dopey and Sleepy?*)

- Vitamin or Mineral Deficiencies
- Sluggish adrenals
- Hypoglycemia (low-blood sugar)
- Excess carbohydrates/sugars
- Allergies
- Anemia
- Poor digestion and malabsorption
- Celiac Sprue disease
- Poor diet
- Side effect of prescription drugs
- Heavy metal toxicity
- Mineral imbalance
- Negative thinking
- Chronic Fatigue Syndrome
- Sluggish thyroid
- Diabetes
- Sluggish liver
- Candida Albicans
- Excessive stress
- Constipation
- Epstein Barr virus
- Insomnia
- Toxic liver or bloodstream
- Hormone imbalance
- Stress
- Estrogen dominance

Diet is major! Eliminate all stimulants which decrease rather than increase energy, including candy, sugar, coffee, tea, soda and junk food. Try to eat 5-9 servings of fresh fruits and veggies a day. Progesterone is also helpful. Exercise moderately a few times a week, for 30 minutes. If you are exhausted after exercise, wait until you regain your health before exercising. Have your doctor check your thyroid.

Recommended supplements for fatigue:
- **Antioxidants (Vitamins A, C, E and selenium)**
- **Magnesium**
- **Vitamin B complex, Folic acid/B12 and Iron (per test results)**
- **Essential oils (Omega-3)**
- **Zinc and Chromium**
- **Ginseng**
- **Natural progesterone supplementation**

Insomnia

There are many reasons for sleep problems. Often sleep problems are related to a decline in estrogen or a combination of estrogen and progesterone deficiencies. Another cause is blood-sugar imbalances. To maintain normal blood-sugar balance, follow the principles in Part 4 of this book.

Drinking too much caffeine or soda a short time before bed is a common cause for a sleepless night, but so is anything else stimulating such as exercising late at night, or experiencing great emotional stress. When appropriate, add some moderate exercise.

Recommended supplements:
- **Calcium and/or Magnesium, Zinc, Chromium and/or Gymnema**
- **Natural progesterone/estrogen supplementation**
- **Vitamin B complex**
- **Essential oils (Omega-3)**
- **Valerian Root or Hops**
- **Liver detoxification program**

Consult with your health professional for a liver detox, and adrenal and thyroid saliva test. Recommendations from the results of these tests can correct the deficiencies related to insomnia. For the person with a serious sleeping problem, a sleep clinic may be recommended.

Stomachaches, Gas and Bloating

People often take digestion for granted. I recently had a client tell me her digestion was fine. However, her dietary history indicated that digestion was her biggest complaint. When I asked her about it she said, "Oh, I have stomachaches frequently, bloating, and constipation, but isn't that normal?"

No, it's not normal, but it is common. We were designed for good digestion and good health.

Americans pop digestive aids like candy and spend millions of dollars a year on laxatives and antacids; yet they continue to suffer from poor digestion and elimination. If these products really "fixed" the problem, why do they still need them? What's the real problem? In his book, *The Mysterious Cause of Illness,*

Dr. Jonn Matsen explains that our stomachs "harden" in response to eating and drinking certain substances. We then think we can eat anything, because we seem to get away with it for a time. Sooner or later, however, digestive problems surface.[47] This is the beginning sign of fatigue and disease.

The first cause of digestive problems is the lack of digestive enzymes and hydrochloric acid (HCl). Anything that hinders your body's ability to digest food causes excess gas and bloating; especially foods that are more difficult to digest (you know, Mexican food!) or more processed such as junk foods and fried foods (of course you never eat these!).

Another reason for gas is the imbalance of friendly to unfriendly bacteria in the body. This also causes yeast infections and urinary tract infections. We need 85% friendly bacteria to 15% unfriendly. Taking some type of acidophilus supplement, often called probiotics, helps with gas.

Anxiety, stress, emotional upsets, antibiotics, and eating too fast can cause gas and bloating. Overeating and some drugs are possible culprits, too.

Recommended supplements:

· **Digestive enzymes and/or Hydrochloric acid (HCl)**
· **Probiotics**
· **Liver detoxification program**
· **Essential oils (Omega-3 fats)**
· **Fiber**

Excessive gas may be a symptom of more serious problems with the colon such as diverticulitis. If these solutions don't help, see your natural health care professional for specific tests.

Gallbladder Problems

Hormone replacement therapy (HRT) may raise a woman's likelihood of developing gallstones. A gallstone can develop when bile, cholesterol, calcium salts and other substances come together to form a mass in the gallbladder. Gallstones often exist without causing symptoms, but surgery is sometimes necessary when the stones cause severe pain.

Researchers studied more than 13,000 middle-aged women who enrolled in the European Prospective Investigation Into Cancer in 1993. Because gallstones are composed primarily of cholesterol, the researchers believe that the use of estrogen could promote an increase in cholesterol in bile that leads to gallstone formation.[48]

Digestive enzyme supplements with high amounts of lipase are particularly helpful for gallbladder problems.

If you've had your gallbladder removed, you need to take bile salts with your meals. Without your gallbladder, your body's ability to store and concentrate bile is impaired, which interferes with fat digestion and proper cholesterol levels. Without bile salts, you may experience fatty acid deficiencies which cause hair, skin and even heart problems. (I use a professional product called Cholacol from Standard Process.)

Additionally, I recommend a liver detoxification program.

Recommended supplements:
- **Digestive enzymes and/or Hydrochloric acid (HCl)**
- **Additional lipase enzymes**
- **Essential oils**
- **Liver detoxification program**

Low Libido (Sex Drive)

I've discovered that for most women, having a low libido is the norm! Men's sex drives aren't as easily decreased. Could this be one of the reasons for so much pornography and infidelity in America? (Besides at our age, most of us women really go to bed to get our beauty sleep!) Estrogen dominance lowers a woman's sex drive, so giving her **more** estrogen will only aggravate the problem. Progesterone is the hormone that increases her sex drive. Progesterone cream is great for this, as evidenced by the stream of men who come in daily to pick up a jar of progesterone cream for their wives!

Women need Omega-3 fats which are required in the pathway of hormone production. So I recommend flaxseed oil or flaxseeds for low libido. Since the adrenals are involved in hormone production, support the adrenals as well.

Recommended supplements for low libido:
· **Natural progesterone supplementation**
· **Flaxseeds or flaxseed oil and adrenal support**

Migraines and Headaches

Migraines indicate inadequate blood supply to the brain, artery constriction and instability of vascular function—either excessive dilation or contraction of blood vessels.

Common lifestyle causes may be unbalanced blood-sugar levels, too little sleep, emotional changes, lack of exercise and changes in barometric pressure.

Common physical causes of migraines are hormone imbalance, vitamin and mineral deficiencies, toxicity, chronic stress, thick blood, and high histamine levels. Most of these can be helped with diet.

I've helped hundreds of women with migraines by just getting them on a progesterone that raised their levels of both progesterone and estrogen naturally. A good protocol includes three months on natural progesterone.

Check the diet to eliminate allergens including: eggs, wheat or dairy, and check additionally for citrus juices, red wine, nitrates in foods, chocolate, aged meats, canned fish, refined sugars, and processed foods. Especially eliminate excess caffeine, soft drinks and MSG.

Recommended supplements:
· **Natural progesterone supplementation**
· **Ginkgo or Vitamin E complex (to thin the blood)**
· **Vitamin B complex (if caused by stress or low blood sugar)**
· **Essential oils (Omega-3)**
· **Magnesium (for relaxation)**
· **Liver detoxification program**

In even more severe cases, I have had to recommend B6 Niacinimide and a liver detoxification program. (See my book, *Why Do I Feel So Lousy?*)

Hormonal Weight Gain

Many women, notice that as they approach menopause, they gain 10-15 extra pounds without changing either their diet or exercise level. Yes, ladies, it's your hormones! Author of *The Menopause Diet,* Dr. Larrian Gillespie explains that in a series of mechanisms following a hot flash, cortisol levels go up which turns off your fat-burning mechanisms.[49]

Weight gain may be linked to a decrease in progesterone which normally keeps fat from being deposited. Additionally, women often become more sedentary or eat more processed foods during this time, both of which will cause weight gain.

A common complaint is weight gain from taking HRT or the Birth Control Pill. I've found that until the woman stops taking the Pill, she will not lose weight easily. Women who are estrogen dominant can gain weight and become fatigued since excess estrogen depresses thyroid and adrenal function.

To lose weight, eat a diet which has foods low on the glycemic index. The glycemic index rates foods on how they affect your blood sugar levels. Refined carbohydrates, such as white breads, pasta and cereals have a higher glycemic index than whole-grain breads, for example. Foods higher on the glycemic index tend to cause weight gain. (For information on weight loss, see my book, *Why Can't I Lose Weight?*)

Starting a walking program can help tremendously. Along with exercise, eat more frequently (every 2-3 hours) to help promote healthy blood sugar levels.

Your body wants to make estrogen from fat and the fat cells in your abdomen are best equipped to produce hormones than fat cells in other places. So gaining a few abdominal pounds is not all that bad. Some good news is that the more fat you have, the less hot flashes and other hormonal imbalances you'll have. Now is not the time to obsess about every calorie and fat gram!

Recommended supplements:

- **Natural progesterone supplementation**
- **Chromium, Magnesium and Zinc**
- **Vitamin B complex (if caused by stress or low blood sugar)**
- **Essential oils (Omega-3)**
- **Thyroid and adrenal support**
- **Liver detoxification program**

Hair Loss

Life is funny. Just when we finally get the right hair style, cut and color, it turns gray and starts to fall out! Talk about a bad hair day!

I've helped dozens of women regrow their hair. There are many causes for hair loss. Here are some I have found:

- Poor diet consisting of too much sugar, junk food
- Not enough protein in diet
- Adrenal stress (physical/emotional stress)
- Low thyroid or other thyroid problems
- Hormone imbalance
- Vitamin deficiencies: B, C or E complex deficiencies
- Mineral deficiencies: zinc, iron
- Toxicity, such as aspartame or toxic mineral such as mercury
- Deficiency of essential fats
- Side effect of certain medications

Get enough protein, fats and minerals in vegetables and fruits. Take hydrochloric acid, without which you can't absorb minerals and digest proteins well.

Recommended supplements:

- **Natural progesterone supplementation**
- **Multiple mineral support**
- **Vitamin B complex (if caused by stress or low blood sugar)**
- **Essential oils (Omega-3 fat)**
- **Thyroid and adrenal support**
- **Liver detoxification program**

Losing hair can be a wake-up call for something serious, so you'll want to work with your natural health professional. Also, see your doctor to rule out any medical problem, (adrenal or thyroid) or if your hair loss is a result of the side effects of certain medications. (Drugs may interfere with the effectiveness of your nutritional supplement and dietary program.)

Let's move on to other sources of hormone problems.

Chapter Eight

Adrenal Stress, Your Liver and Progesterone

"Never mind the hot flashes," one of my clients recently said. "I'd just like to go a day without weeping and sobbing!"

Your adrenal glands help manage stress. However, when we live in continual stress, our adrenal glands become so tired, they can't handle stress or female hormones properly.

Think about the average woman's life. Most of her waking hours are spent taking care of her house, her children and her husband's needs. Many of these women also work part- or full-time. By the end of the day, she's spent time taking care of everyone but herself!

Your hormonal balance reflects your health. If your adrenals are exhausted, you'll have hormone problems. If your liver is toxic, you'll have hormone problems. If your blood-sugar levels are off, you'll have hormone problems.

Symptoms of Stress

We don't always recognize stress as it occurs and we may not even be aware of how much stress we are under. We may think we are "just handling it," but our adrenal glands are quietly becoming exhausted. Here are symptoms of stress:

- Fatigue
- Anger
- Headaches
- Lowered resistance
- Low-blood sugar
- Insomnia
- Cravings
- Dizziness
- Depression
- Aches and pain
- Anxiety
- Low blood pressure
- Weight gain

After years of stress, a woman may experience adrenal insufficiency which, according to Dr. Lee, causes hormone imbalance including these symptoms:[50]

- Irregular menstrual cycles
- Anovulatory periods
- Fibrocystic breasts
- Infertility

Additionally, once her adrenals become weak, her thyroid gland slows down to compensate. This can cause low blood pressure and weight gain. These are not cases of estrogen deficiency, but rather progesterone deficiency.

Marla came to me saying, "My night sweats were so bad, I couldn't sleep, I gained weight and my joints were hurting. I took the adrenal supplements that Lorrie recommended and all of these symptoms left."

Many women have taken diet pills which have stressed both their adrenal glands and thyroid. So many "female issues" such as anxiety, panic attacks, inability to lose weight, hair loss, and fatigue are due to exhausted adrenal glands.

My assistant, Lori, suffered from many classic symptoms of General Anxiety Disorder before she came to see me. She experienced tingling in the feet, hands and lips, hair-loss, never-ending muscle tension, fatigue, dizzy spells, heart palpitations, skin sensitivity and general feelings of fear and anxiety. Behind all of these symptoms were nutritional imbalances that were corrected with a balanced diet, nutritional supplements, exercise and stress management.

Recommended Supplements for Stress:

- **Antioxidants (Vitamins A, C, E and selenium)**
- **Magnesium**
- **Vitamin B complex**
- **Essential oils**
- **Eleuthero Root (Siberian Ginseng by Medi-Herb)**
- **Panax Ginseng and/or Licorice Root**
- **Gymnema and/or Chromium GTF**
- **Withania (Ashwaganda by Medi-Herb)**

(I use Medi-Herb natural herbs which you can only buy through a licensed, health professional, not over-the-counter.)

An excellent way to check both thyroid and adrenal levels is through saliva hormone testing for both adrenals and thyroid. (See my book, *Why Am I So Grumpy, Dopey and Sleepy?* for additional details on thyroid and adrenal health.)

How's Your Liver?

Earlier I mentioned how easy it is for women to become estrogen dominant. It's the liver's job to "clear" the excess estrogens, so they won't become toxic and raise her estrogen levels. A common symptom of liver sluggishness is bloating before or during her cycle. So, female hormone balance depends on a woman having a healthy liver!

In her most fascinating book, *The Healthy Liver and Bowel Book,* (great bathroom reading!) Australian Doctor Sandra Cabot lists the many, many symptoms associated with liver dysfunction. They include:[51]

• **Abnormal metabolism of fats** including cellulite, weight gain, fat around the middle, pot belly, high cholesterol and triglycerides.

• **Digestive problem**s including reflux, gallstones, nausea, irritable bowel and pain in the liver.

• **Blood sugar problems** including cravings for sugar.

• **Nervous system problems** including depression, mood swings and foggy brain.

• **Immune dysfunction** including allergies, skin rashes, Chronic Fatigue Syndrome, and Fibromyalgia.

• **Hormonal imbalance** including menopausal symptoms and PMS.

Nausea, Morning Sickness and the Liver

Some women become nauseous around their cycles and many become nauseous when they become pregnant.

I recently saw a book on morning sickness and how to handle it, which gave suggestions such as eating saltine crackers. While I think the information could be helpful, I was surprised that it never talked about how to **prevent** it. Everyone thinks it's normal to have nausea, but nausea is a signal of weak digestion and a congested liver.

I often find that this is the case with many books, especially when written by medical experts. They are excellent at labeling and describing the symptoms and/or suggesting mechanical devices or drugs to treat the symptoms, yet rarely talk about how to prevent or heal them.

This is because nutritional deficiencies and biochemical imbalances affecting organ and gland function are the missing links that are usually over-looked. You can prevent nausea by taking enzymes, cleansing the liver, and eating a healthy diet six months to a year **before** you get pregnant. For nausea, I recommend Vitamin B6, magnesium and Phosfood Liquid® (from Standard Process®) which eliminates the sludge trapped in your gallbladder which causes nausea and vomiting. Drink 10 drops in 1/4 to 1 cup of water as needed.

Cleansing the Liver

I've supervised hundreds of cleansing programs with my menopausal clients. One client said, "I'm amazed at how much better I feel after following Lorrie's liver cleanse. Not only do I have more energy, but all of my symptoms of menopause are gone—especially the night sweats, hot flashes, and sleeping problems."

Cathy said, "I came to Lorrie because when my doctor put me on a "natural" triple estrogen, I gained 15 pounds in a month! Nothing fit me. I couldn't sleep at night and I had no sex drive. I did Lorrie's liver cleanse program and in three weeks, I lost all 15 pounds and my sex drive is normal."

Both clients followed a cleanse which I discuss in my book, *Why Do I Feel So Lousy?* Also, taking acidophilus (found in yogurt) helps the liver to detoxify toxic estrogen.

Raise Your Progesterone Levels

The reason so many women in this country are progesterone deficient is that unlike estrogen, there are no food sources of progesterone, yet there are many cultural, lifestyle, environmental and dietary factors that increase estrogen levels, causing "estrogen dominance."

There are two ways to increase your levels of progesterone. You can use: 1) Herbs, such as Chaste Tree; and 2) Natural progesterone supplements.

Chaste Tree

Chaste Tree is a common herb that helps your body to make progesterone which has been used for centuries. It has several names, but each of these is the same herb: Chaste Tree, Chasteberry or Vitex. I recommend the herb Chaste Tree from Medi-Herb especially for younger women since it's effective for regulating cycles.

Sources of Progesterone

There are three ways to take natural progesterone: trans-dermally (a cream you rub on the skin), sublingually (under the tongue) and orally (a pill). Oral progesterone isn't as effective since the liver de-activates 50-90% of the oral hormones; so larger doses must be given which overworks the liver. I prefer and have experience with using the cream.

Studies on the Cream

I've seen more than 7,000 women in the past several years and I've found that my progesterone cream is one of the best supplements for most of them. For example, when a woman comes in with severe estrogen dominance, the cream works extremely fast to eliminate depression, aches and pain, and other symptoms of estrogen dominance. Then we have some time to get started working on her diet, nutrition and exercise program. Often, I recommend the cream short-term.

Conclusions of a study reported in *Fertility and Sterility* said that: trans-dermal progesterone is well absorbed; trans-dermal progesterone reduced breast cell proliferation; and trans-dermal progesterone, administered monthly, reduced the risk of breast cancers.[52]

The creams are preferred over the patch or pills, since the delivery bypasses the already overworked liver.

Most hormonal imbalances are commonly due to progesterone deficiency. Compare symptoms in the following chart which I compiled and rewrote from Raquel Martin's book, *The Estrogen Alternative.*[53]

Symptoms of Estrogen Dominance	Benefits of Progesterone Supplementation
• Weight gain	• Weight loss
• Insomnia	• Restful sleep
• Female cancer risk	• Helps prevent female cancers
• Depression	• Helps prevent depression
• Fluid retention (bloating)	• Helps water balance
• Thyroid imbalance	• Assists thyroid hormone action
• Blood clots	• Normalizes blood clotting
• Migraine headaches	• Prevents migraines
• Risk of miscarriage	• Prevents miscarriages
• Cramping	• Relieves cramping
• Elevated blood pressure	• Regulates blood pressure
• Acne	• Helps skin
• Irregular menstrual flow	• Normalizes cycles
• Restrains bone loss	• Helps grow bone

Profit Over Health?

Dr. John Lee wrote that research on natural progesterone has in the past two decades been essentially nonexistent. He reported that the pharmaceutical companies take perfectly good natural hormones that our bodies know and can use and alter them, creating synthetic compounds (Provera) with similar hormonal effects but toxic side effects.[54]

The misunderstanding between natural progesterone and progestins is common, but there is a great difference: Natural progesterone has no known side effects when used properly, while those of synthetic progestins, synthetic progesterone, commonly prescribed and sold as Provera has high risks associated with it: Birth defects, fluid retention, epilepsy, migraines, asthma, cardiac or kidney dysfunction and depression, pulmonary embolism, and menstrual irregularities.

Who Should Raise Their Progesterone Levels?

Most women benefit from using natural progesterone, but especially any woman who has taken estrogen replacement therapy or the Pill, has PMS, is trying to get pregnant, has had a miscarriage, or suffers from depression. Any woman who has had a hysterectomy really needs progesterone.[55]

Results of Progesterone Therapy

I've seen some wonderful results from women using progesterone cream. Here is a testimony from a woman I interviewed named Cynthia Drasler:

> I have been using a hormone cream since February of 1997, with dramatic results. I had fibrocystic breast disease for 22 years. After 3 months of using this cream, my fibrocystic breast condition was gone. I was amazed and delighted. My only regret about natural progesterone is that I didn't know about it twenty years ago.

Another client named Karen said, "I love using the cream! My periods only last a few days, and I no longer have fibrous tumors or breast tenderness—my breasts used to be lumpy like cottage cheese. I no longer have hot flashes or mood swings. I used to have headaches so bad that I thought I was dying! I can't take estrogen, even in the mildest form. Don't ever take the cream away from me, because it works!"

Monica said, "I had a lot of cramps before if I didn't take Ibuprofen, it would hurt. Because of the cream, during this last cycle, I haven't had to take any medications. It's a miracle."

Should I Get My Hormones Tested?

Before supplementing with progesterone, I would suggest that you have your hormone levels checked.

Doctors order blood tests. However, they rarely check progesterone levels, and symptoms can be felt even though the tests reveal that her hormones are within "normal." If a woman's estrogen levels come out lower than "normal," doctors recommend estrogen (which causes estrogen dominance) and often ignore progesterone. The saliva test measures the most active part of the hormones, so they are more accurate than blood tests. See your health professional regarding which hormone saliva tests are best for your needs.

Most saliva hormone test kits measure estrogen, progesterone and testosterone and are easy to understand. You'll have to spit into small plastic containers and send them to the lab. Don't brush your teeth or eat or drink anything one hour before your sample. Be sure to read the directions and return your samples quickly so they don't spoil in the mail. I suggest overnight mail.

While I've had excellent results with recommending the cream, trans-dermal progesterone is more difficult to monitor, and it's possible to get too much progesterone. Long-term use and too much progesterone can possibly lead to depression. That's why you need to work with your natural healthcare professional to get the best source of progesterone.

Another important test to assist in hormone balancing is a Tissue Mineral Hair Analysis. Hormones are the messengers; minerals are the receivers. If you have mineral deficiencies, excesses or imbalances, it can affect your hormone levels. Therefore, sometimes both the saliva hormone test and the tissue mineral hair analysis are recommended.

How Do I Use It?

Hormone expert Dr. John Lee recommended progesterone cream that is applied trans-dermally which means "across the skin." The advantage is that it bypasses the liver and goes to specific receptor sites where progesterone is needed. That means it helps immediately, which gives us time to help one of the causes for hormone imbalance—a sluggish liver!

The general way to use progesterone cream is to apply 1/4 teaspoon twice a day. Don't try to "rush" the process by using too much cream; it generally takes 3 months to raise your progesterone level. Apply the cream on the soft-tissue parts of your skin such as the inside of your wrists, on your tummy, or on the underside of your arm (not where you put your deodorant!). There are different ways to use the cream according to where you are in your cycles. You will want to work with your health care professional to get the best results.

If you spot a little or experience a double cycle, there is generally no cause for alarm. If you start using the progesterone cream and you begin to notice symptoms such as breast swelling, water retention, headaches or insomnia, this happens because the progesterone temporarily increases the sensitivity of estrogen receptors, which means you might have symptoms of estrogen dominance **temporarily.** However, see your health professional for help with the temporary symptoms as your body finds balance.

Progesterone cream can help your thyroid, so if you are taking thyroid supplements, you may want to discuss weaning off of them with your doctor.

Most women have immediate benefits; but I've had a client who took three full months before she saw results. Women who have had a complete hysterectomy will need to use additional estrogen, in a natural form as well.

In all of these years, I've only had one woman who was extremely toxic and reacted strongly to the cream. We had to back up and help her to cleanse her liver.

Give Progesterone Time to Work

Please give yourself a minimum of three cycles on progesterone to rebalance your hormones, especially if you are trying to get pregnant. Many women have reported instant results and relief, while others may take a few weeks or months before these benefits are seen. Women get better results if they are also following a healthy diet.

Used properly, progesterone supplements are incredible with no side effects. However, I've found six things that can interfere with the effectiveness of natural progesterone.

1. She is not progesterone deficient; most of the time this would include small, underweight women who are truly estrogen deficient.

2. She has self-prescribed and is using an ineffective source of progesterone.

3. If she's using the cream, she's probably using too much. Dr. Lee taught that the cream must be used the way a woman would normally produce progesterone, and only during the proper times of the month. For example, it's really important that non-cycling women take a break from the cream at least 6 days a month. For these women, taking the cream all month without any breaks will only cause it to be eventually ineffective.

I've heard women teach other women to just "slap it on" their skin any time there is a hot flash. That's not a good idea. Dr. Lee taught that the closer you can get to how your own body produces progesterone, the better. Occassionally, women can overuse the hormone cream. Symptoms of excess progesterone include: bloating, constipation, sleepiness, and mild depression. (There are many, many steps to taking progesterone cream properly. Use the cream only under professional guidance.)

4. She's not handling stress well.

5. She doesn't get the sleep that she needs.

6. She's not changing her diet to that of a healthy, whole-foods diet that supports adrenal balance and normal blood-sugar levels. She may need a liver detoxification program.

Pregnancy and Progesterone

Because progesterone deficiency can cause infertility and even miscarriages, many women have been able to become pregnant within three months of using progesterone supplementation. I always recommend that if she can, she wait until this 3-month cycle so she is sure that she won't miscarry because of progesterone deficiency. The healthier the woman is before pregnancy, the easier her pregnancy and delivery will be. I also recommend support for the adrenal glands and a liver detox before a woman becomes pregnant.

If you have been using progesterone and you become pregnant, don't stop using it abruptly. Doing so will signal the body to shed the uterine lining, and possibly induce a miscarriage. Continue to use progesterone to prevent the menstrual shedding until the third month of the pregnancy at which time you can taper your progesterone with the help of your natural healthcare professional.

Infertile women benefit from folic acid and B12, which I recommend prior to pregnancy as well as during pregnancy. Food sources (or whole-food supplements) containing all of the vitamins, the B complex, vitamin E and zinc are also important for fertility. I also recommend taking iron and calcium prior to pregnancy as well as during pregnancy. While progesterone helps with post-partum depression, if she is breastfeeding, she should not use the cream.

See your natural health care professional for help regarding progesterone, and to get a whole-food prenatal protocol and discuss any special nutritional or dietary factor so you can ensure a healthy pregnancy, delivery and lactation.

How Long Should I Use Progesterone?

If a woman strengthens her adrenal glands, detoxes her liver, and follows a healthy eating plan, she can probably maintain normal hormone levels without any natural estrogen or progesterone supplementation. Otherwise, she should stay on the cream until her adrenals are strong.

I work with each client individually to determine if and how long they should use the natural progesterone cream.

Estrogen Dominance and Disease

Since estrogen dominance causes hormonal imbalances, I've helped women eliminate hot flashes, handle PMS symptoms, eliminate breast tenderness, normalize cycles, and eliminate depression by using progesterone cream. But natural progesterone helps serious conditions, too.

Estrogen causes cells in the breast and endometrium to multiply. Without a balance of (natural) progesterone to estrogen, estrogen overproduces breast cells and uterine tissues and causes uterine lining build-up. This can lead to fibroids, cysts, endometriosis, fibrocystic breasts, and breast cancer. Natural progesterone supplementation is essential. Dr. John Lee's books discuss these conditions in detail, but in this book I want to show you the connection between estrogen dominance and these conditions. Work with your natural health professional for specific nutritional protocols.

Fibroids

Fibroids are the most common benign tumors in Western women; one out of five women has them. They can range in size from the size of an orange to a football. The rate of growth is slow, but they can grow when a woman is under stress. Estrogen causes fibroids to grow, which is why having a hysterectomy or the decreasing levels of estrogen at menopause usually cause them to shrink. (See your doctor.)

Fibroids can cause pelvic pain, heavy bleeding at menstruation, anemia, constipation, hemorrhoids, or bladder problems. Women without children often have fibroids more than women with children, because of high estrogen levels. Take progesterone, flaxseeds, and Vitamin E complex. I highly recommend you work with a healthcare professional.

Ovarian Cysts

Both ovarian cysts and Polycystic Ovarian Syndrome (PCOS) are linked to decreasing levels of progesterone or estrogen dominance. Birth Control Pills are commonly used to suppress the cycle which may shrink the cyst. However, this only treats the symptom, but not the cause. (See the discussion in Chapter 4 about the side effects of the Pill.) If you have irregular or missed cycles, check with your health professional about using a supplement or herbs for producing more progesterone which helps re-establish the normal hormonal cycle.

Common symptoms of PCOS are: high testosterone levels which may also cause weight gain, facial hair growth, high insulin levels, infertility and acne. Exercising and eliminating refined sugars and refined carbohydrates help lower insulin levels and which also helps with PCOS.

Endometriosis

Symptoms include pain, infertility and lack of ovulation. This type of pain is found in the lower back, vagina and lower abdomen. While there is no definitive cause, it's commonly believed that estrogen dominance and progesterone deficiency are involved and other factors include a high animal meat diet, alcohol, sugar and caffeine.

For pain, the herb Cramp Bark is recommended. Herbs which assist in promoting progesterone production, such as Chaste Tree or natural progesterone are recommended. Additionally, take extra antioxidants (vitamins A, C, E and selenium), Echinacea and wheat germ. Eating a healthy, whole-foods diet is highly recommended.

Fibrocystic Breast Tissue

This is the development of lumpy breasts or benign breast lumps, which range from very small to golf ball size. Often referred to as Fibrocystic Breast Disease, they don't cause cancer or predispose us to breast cancer. Even healthy breasts are still somewhat lumpy especially if women drink coffee, eat meat and dairy, and have high stress levels.

Benign cysts don't happen after menopause unless a woman takes synthetic hormone replacement which raises estrogen to a higher than normal level. During natural menopause, fibrous growths usually shrink.

I recommend vitamin E, flaxseed oil or Omega-3 fat from fish, and the natural hormone progesterone cream. Also, adding extra fiber helps your body to excrete toxic estrogen. Iodine can also reduce the sensitivity to estrogen.

Breast Cancer

One in nine women will be diagnosed with breast cancer in her lifetime. Breast cancer is second only to lung cancer as the most common cause of cancer death in American women.

Estrogen dominance, HRT and the Pill are the biggest causes of breast cancer. High levels of estrogen can lead to cell growth. Dietary links to high estrogen levels are excessive intake of animal fats, caffeine and refined sugars, obesity, insufficient nutrients for the liver to clear estrogen, and lack of essential antioxidants and essential fats. You will need to work with a health care professional who has both training and experience in breast cancer. Don't self medicate. Eating a healthy diet, rich in fruits and vegetables is vital. Follow a liver cleanse and take whole-food supplements and a green food supplement.

Exercise has been shown to be one of the best ways to prevent breast cancer, since exercise can help lower estrogen. A moderate 45 minutes five days a week are recommended.

A common medical treatment for breast cancer is Tamoxifen which is a drug approved by the FDA to reduce the risk of breast cancer. But according to Dr. Arnot, author of *The Breast Cancer Prevention Diet,* some people fear that the drug only delays breast cancer, rather than entirely prevents it.[56]

Researcher Sherrill Sellman reports that while the initial findings of Tamoxifen's role in breast cancer treatment were promising, as with so many synthetic drugs, further research shows grave concerns including: hot flashes, vaginal discharge, eye damage, blood clots, asthma, vocal cord changes, liver cancer, liver disease, and endometrial cancer.[57]

More than 600,000 Americans take chemo at their doctor's recommendations. But is it safe, effective and necessary? If you are thinking about this therapy, I highly recommend *Questioning Chemotherapy* by Dr. Ralph W. Moss. Dr. Moss is an internationally-acclaimed science writer with a twenty-year career writing about cancer. In this book, Moss closely examines such issues as chemo success and failure rates for over 50 types of cancer as well as if it works and how to counter side effects. I also highly recommend Dr. John Lee's book, *What Your Doctor May Not Tell You About Breast Cancer,* Dr. Patrick Quillin's book, *Beating Cancer With Nutrition,* and Maureen Salaman's book, *The Cancer Answer*.

Cervical Dysplasia

Cervical dysplasia is caused by estrogen dominance. While dysplasia means abnormal cell growth, this does not mean that it's cancer. Since there is a concern that it could become cancerous, having a Pap smear which can identify cell changes is recommended. Symptoms are a persistent discharge from the vagina which may create itching or burning anywhere from cervix to vulva. The Birth Control Pill is linked to cervical cancer, possibly since the Pill causes vitamin deficiencies.

Conventional medical care involves burning or freezing the cervix. Folic acid is essential for protecting DNA from damage, which is more likely with estrogen dominance. In addition to a better diet, nutritional recommendations are acidophilus, zinc, the B complex, Echinacea and antioxidants.

Estrogen dominance is linked to not only discomforts of hormone balance, but also serious disease. I've found that using natural progesterone helps in nearly every case.

Let's now move to Part 4, eating for your hormone health.

PART FOUR

Eating for Hormone Health

Chapter Nine

Nutrition, Diet and Hormones

Diet, nutrition and weight loss books are popular, especially written by celebrities—you know, people whose income comes from staying in shape and working out for four hours a day! And if they gain a pound, they can easily afford plastic surgery to have it removed!

Regular exercise is vital for good health, but also for relief from hot flashes, improved heart function, improved circulation, reduced blood pressure, improved ability to deal with stress, and increase in energy and endurance. Exercise also reduces risk of osteoporosis. (See *Why Am I So Grumpy, Dopey and Sleepy?* or *Why Can't I Lose Weight?*)

Hormone health requires all three parts:
• Natural progesterone/estrogen supplementation as required
• Regular exercise
• Proper nutrition and appropriate supplements

The better a woman eats, the less negative symptoms of PMS and menopause she will experience. Women can't be healthy on a junk food diet!

Most of my clients have been amazed at how much better they feel after making a few changes in their diets which support their blood-sugar levels, their adrenals, and the ability of their liver to remove toxic estrogens.

The best diet for hormone health revolves around whole, "real" plant foods such as fruits and vegetables which contain lots of cancer-fighting nutrients and fiber, along with lean protein, essential fats and complex carbohydrates.

What to Eat and Why

1. Fruits and vegetables are rich sources of phytochemicals and phytoestrogens, which help protect against breast cancer and other diseases.

Bioflavonoid antioxidants found in berries and carotenoid antioxidants (vitamins C and A), such as orange, yellow and red fruits and vegetables are great. For example, have blueberries on your cereal or in your protein drink, or eat an orange for breakfast; have a salad with leafy greens, carrots or tomatoes at lunch; and have steamed broccoli and a sweet potato for dinner. Fruits and vegetables are so protective that the National Cancer Institute recommends that we eat nine servings of fruits and vegetables a day. Top antioxidant foods are: Garlic, kale, spinach, Brussels sprouts, alfalfa sprouts, broccoli, beets, red bell pepper and onions.[58]

Eating the whole fruit (orange or apple) is preferable to drinking the juice (orange juice or apple juice) because of the high amount of concentrated sugars in the juice.

Probably one of the best additions to any woman's diet is that of cruciferous vegetables, you know, the ones that none of your teenagers want to eat! They include broccoli, cauliflower, bok choy, Brussels sprouts, cabbage, kale, and so on. One of the ingredients in these veggies is indole-3 carbinol, which can increase good estrogen and decrease the bad estrogen as reported in a study in *The Journal of the National Cancer Institute.* According to Dr. Arnot, author of *The Breast Cancer Prevention Diet,* cruciferous vegetables decreased breast cancer risk by 40 percent in a Wisconsin study.[59]

2. Fiber-rich foods are important since they can help to lower estrogen levels. Plant foods are the only source of fiber which helps to eliminate toxins, lower cholesterol and balance blood-sugar levels. In addition to fruits and vegetables, other good sources of fiber include nuts, seeds, whole grains and beans.

Black beans, lentils and kidney beans are good sources of fiber, phytoestrogens and protein. They are easy to use in recipes and excellent for diabetics. (Use a digestive aid such as a digestive enzyme or Beano.)

According to Dr. Arnot, soy beans may protect against breast cancer by reducing levels of estrogen.[60] Also, eating soy vegetable protein stimulates the liver to rid the body of excess estrogen.

However, soy isn't a miracle food, and not everyone can digest soy products. Soy hinders thyroid function and it contains compounds that block absorption of minerals such as zinc. Additionally, soy is often grown with the use of heavy pesticides.

Yet there are benefits to eating soy, so to find a balance, I recommend eating traditional, organically-grown sources of fermented soy products: tempeh, which has a texture similar to beef; miso, which is a paste used for flavoring soups; and tamari (natural soy sauce). Tofu, while not fermented, is a traditional source of soy as well.

While processed soy products are popular (soy candy bars, cookies, burgers, soy drinks, soy protein bars, and so on), they don't have the same cancer-fighting benefits of natural, organic soy. Dr. Lee believes that soybean toxins are more concentrated in these products and they may do more harm than good. Additionally, several of my vegetarian clients who were living on an all soy protein-based diet had the most trouble losing weight.

3. Whole grains such as oatmeal, barley, brown rice, millet, rye and spelt are also good sources of fiber. Whole wheat flour and flour products are okay if there is no allergy to wheat. Limit carbohydrate servings to 3-4 daily, and only eat the whole-grain carbohydrates.[61]

4. Essential fatty acids in the form of extra virgin olive oil, flaxseed oil, salmon, tuna, almonds, and Evening Primrose Oil all help hormone balance. Flaxseeds are the richest plant source of Omega-3 fatty acids. Grind up flaxseeds fresh and take 1-2 tablespoons daily.

5. Lean protein, especially fish (salmon, tuna, mackerel, trout), organically grown lean red meat, and poultry are all important for hormone balance. While excess red meat consumption isn't good, most of my female clients don't eat enough protein, which causes loss of muscle tone, hair loss and a weakened immune system. Take digestive enzymes.

6. Drink plenty of pure water; one half your body weight in ounces.

What to Avoid and Why

Americans sure eat a lot of processed, artificial foods. In fact, I've often wondered if they continue eating these artificial foods, how much longer before they are declared an artificial life form?

1. Avoid caffeine, coffee, soft drinks, black tea and chocolate. I know, you think chocolate is good for you, but not when it's loaded with sugar! Caffeine depletes the B vitamins and is linked to anxiety and mood swings.

Most women with hormone imbalance also experience adrenal fatigue. It's natural to want coffee when you're tired since any type of caffeine stimulates the adrenal glands. However, drinking more coffee makes you even more tired! Additionally, forcing the adrenal glands to produce hormones causes a higher level of blood sugar and insulin as well. Dr. John Lee said that coffee raises estrogen because it is highly sprayed with pesticides which are xenohormones.[62]

2. Avoid excessive sugar, carbonated beverages and alcohol. Tired women usually crave sugar as well. Sugar also stimulates the adrenal glands and increases glucose and serotonin levels in the brain. Serotonin is a "feel-good" chemical, so eating sugar is a quick way to feel good, but the resultant hormone imbalance isn't worth it!

Refined, white processed sugar not only contains no nutrition, but when you eat it, it actually causes vitamin and mineral deficiencies. Years ago, I heard cancer authority Dr. Patrick Quillin say that one serving of a sugary snack or sugar-laden soda can depress your immune system for the next 6-8 hours. **Sugar causes weight gain, adrenal and thyroid fatigue and insulin resistance.** Soda, including diet soda, leaches calcium from bones and diet sodas often contain Aspartame. (Aspartame is a chemical sweetener in sugar substitutes and gum, which is known to cause brain damage.[63]) The herb stevia is a healthy, natural substitute.

I use whole-food nutritional supplements as a therapy to help women lower their insulin levels and eliminate sugar and carbohydrate cravings. Ask your heath professional about chromium, zinc, magnesium and the herb, Gymnema.

3. Avoid processed carbohydrates. This is many women's major food groups! This includes foods made with white flour: cakes, cookies, cereal, bagels, breads, and pastas. While labeled "low-fat," our body converts them into fat.

In Dr. Arnot's book, *The Breast Cancer Prevention Diet*, four out of his twelve cancer-prevention steps include lowering sugar in the blood: Lower insulin levels, drop glucose overload, increase fiber and limit alcohol. Dr. Arnot cites several studies that link high-insulin levels to breast cancer. He recommends that the next time you have blood work, ask your doctor to include an insulin level check. The normal range is from 79 to 190. Women who eat high-fat, low-fiber diets are apt to have high insulin levels.[64]

4. Reduce or eliminate dairy products. Hormone expert Sherrill Sellman says that contrary to advertising, dairy is one of the worst foods a woman can eat for hormone balance since consuming dairy can increase symptoms of PMS such as swelling, cramping and breast tenderness.[65]

If you must drink milk, realize there are consequences. Dr. John Lee suggests that if you drink milk, get it from cows that are not given bovine growth hormone, known as rBGH, which forces the cow into producing higher quantities of milk. These hormones contain estrogenic factors which fatten the cows up, but are considered by Dr. Lee to be xenohormones.[66]

Dairy products also contain arachidonic acid which can worsen cramps. Dairy products are also high in saturated fats and often are an allergen, and can be difficult to digest.

5. Avoid saturated fat in the form of red meat. Dr. Lee reports that pesticides (chemical estrogens) in the grain fed to livestock are concentrated in the fat of the red meat that we eat. Whenever possible, buy only organic or free-range, hormone-free meat, chicken and dairy products.[67]

According to Dr. Arnot, while red meat eaters showed a 25% increase in the breast cancer rate, all meats could be of lower risk if they are marinated and not grilled over an open fire. Grilling can introduce a potent carcinogen (cancer-causing agent.)[68]

6. Avoid hydrogenated oils (peanut butter, margarine, Crisco), all fried foods, and processed vegetable oils. The processing of these fats changes a normal fat (cis-fatty acid) into what is now called a damaged or trans-fats. Trans-fats are now known to cause a higher cancer and heart disease risk according to Dr. John Lee. Most trans-fats are labeled as hydrogenated or partially hydrogenated oils.[69]

Additionally, the percentage of different types of fats in our diets has changed dramatically over the last century. There are two main types of fats, Omega 6 and Omega-3. Dr. Arnot reports that our Western diet contains up to 20 times as many Omega-6 as Omega-3 fats, or a 20:1 ratio. A healthier ratio should be closer to 4:1.[70]

For years, Americans were told to give up saturated fats for these Omega-6 polyunsaturated fats. Unfortunately, average American women eat 500 times the amount of Omega-6 than is considered healthy.[71]

The American Health Foundation theorizes that Omega-6 fats contribute to the spread of cancer, whereas Omega-3 fats suppress cancer growth.[72] Specific Omega-6 fats to avoid include: hydrogenated corn oil, soybean oil, safflower oil, peanut oil, cottonseed oil, and margarine.

How to Eat

Breakfast is still your most important meal, especially when it comes to female hormone balance and weight control. Eating regular meals, every two to three hours, keeps your blood sugar and insulin levels normal, helps your body handle stress, and helps you lose weight. Dieting and skipping meals only causes further hormone imbalance! Yet overeating raises both estrogen and insulin.

Eat a semi-vegetarian diet, with lots of fresh fruits and vegetables, lean protein, small servings of complex carbohydrates and some good fat! You can make almost any diet healthy if you follow those guidelines. Don't forget to drink plenty of pure water.

A quick and easy breakfast is a protein rich, whey-based shake. Have a large salad with protein at lunch, and a lean protein, vegetables and a complex carbohydrate for dinner.

Sample Meal Plans

Breakfast (Choose One)

1. **Protein Drink**

   1-2 scoops whey protein

   1 Tbs. freshly ground flaxseeds or 1 tsp. flaxseed oil

   Fruit (blueberries, strawberries, banana, peaches, and so on)

   1 cup water or rice milk

2. Oatmeal or Oat Bran (with small amount of protein like an egg or cottage cheese)

3. Poached eggs with one slice of whole grain toast and butter.

   Herbal tea or water

Lunch Choose from a large vegetable salad, animal or vegetable protein (such as beans, legumes, or tempeh) and a complex carbohydrate.

1. Chicken Caesar Salad with one slice of whole-grain bread.

2. Tuna fish salad on whole-grain bread with lettuce, tomato and cucumber. A mixture of flaxseed oil or olive oil and 1/4 cup apple cider vinegar makes a nice dressing.

3. Chickpea salad with carrots and tomatoes on green leafy vegetables with lemon juice, garlic and olive oil dressing.

Dinner

1. Bean chili with a green salad, olive oil or flaxseed oil dressing and three whole-grain crackers.

2. Grilled chicken breast, steamed broccoli and cauliflower with lemon butter seasoning, and baked sweet potato.

3. Grilled Salmon, steamed asparagus spears and carrots, and ½ cup brown rice with 1/2 tsp. flaxseed oil or butter.

Herbal tea or water

Recommended Snacks or Mini-Meals

· ½ cup cottage cheese with ground flaxseeds and fruit
· ½ cup non-fat yogurt with fruit
· Whey protein drink or whey protein bar
· 10 raw almonds, pistachio nuts or cashews
· Raw vegetable sticks
· 2 Wasa bread crackers with 1 slice natural cheese
· 2 Kavli Crispbread with chicken strips and Dijon mustard
· Tuna fish on whole-grain crackers
· 1/4 cup Macadamia nuts

- 1 ounce cashew butter, almond butter or peanut butter on 1 whole grain cracker.
- 1 ounce string cheese, or Feta cheese, or Swiss cheese, or Mozzarella cheese, or white cheese with 3-4 whole grain crackers or one piece of fruit.

Nutritional Supplements

Here is a general nutritional protocol for hormone balance, followed by a recap of the supplements listed in this book. See your natural healthcare professional for nutritional testing. (For information on how to buy supplements, see my book, *Why Do I Need Whole Food Supplements?*)

1. A digestive enzyme supplement.

2. A whole-food multiple vitamin/mineral. (I use Standard Process.) Synthetic vitamins are toxic to the liver and create further stress.

3. A whole-food antioxidant (includes vitamins A, C, E and the mineral selenium). Grapeseed and pycnogenol are 50 to 100 times stronger than vitamins C and E.

4. Calcium/magnesium supplement or other bone-building formula. (Have your natural healthcare professional perform a tissue Hair Mineral Analysis.)

5. Essential oils which contain essential fatty acids important in making prostaglandins for proper hormone function.

6. Adrenal support or herbs, including Licorice root or Siberian ginseng. Also helpful are Vitamin C, E, and B complex and Folic/B12.

7. Liver Detox. I like to use Standard Process SP Cleanse. (For further information, see my book entitled, *Why Do I Feel So Lousy?*)

Supplements for Your Heart
- **Garlic and Ginkgo**
- **Magnesium/calcium**
- **Vitamin B, C and E complex**
- **Essential oils (Omega-3 fats)**
- **Hawthorne**
- **Regular exercise and stress management**

Supplements for Preventing Alzheimer's

- Antioxidants (Vitamins A, C, E and the mineral selenium)
- Essential oils (Omega-3 fats)
- Circulatory support (Ginkgo and Vitamin E complex)
- Nerve support (Vitamin B complex)

Supplements for Preventing Osteoporosis

- Hydrochloric acid
- Magnesium/calcium/manganese
- Vitamins D and K
- Essential oils (Omega-3 fats)
- Natural progesterone supplementation
- Support digestion and thyroid

Supplements for Hot Flashes

- Natural progesterone supplementation
- Black Cohosh or Dong Quai
- Sage or ginseng
- Red Clover
- Chaste Tree
- Flaxseeds (ground fresh)

Supplements for Food Cravings

- Sugar cravings: Chromium GTF, Zinc, or Gymnema
- Chocolate cravings: Magnesium
- Salt cravings: Use Celtic sea salt from your health food store

Supplements for Skin Problems

- Natural progesterone supplementation
- Vitamin A complex
- Zinc
- Acidophilus supplement and digestive enzymes
- Liver/body detoxification
- Essential fats (Omega-3)

Supplements for Anxiety & Heart Palpitations

- Magnesium
- B complex and Valerian Root

Supplements for Depression
- Natural progesterone supplementation
- Vitamin B complex and Folic acid/B12
- Essential oils (Omega-3)
- Ginkgo/ginseng
- St. John's Wort
- Probiotics and liver detoxification

Supplements for Memory Loss
- Essential oils (Omega-3)
- Vitamin B complex and Folic acid/B12
- Ginkgo to improve circulation and boost memory
- Ginseng for alertness, memory and concentration
- Probiotics and liver detoxification

Supplements for Fatigue
- Antioxidants (Vitamins A, C, E and selenium)
- Magnesium
- Vitamin B complex, Folic acid/B12 and Iron (per test results)
- Essential oils (Omega-3)
- Zinc and chromium
- Ginseng
- Natural progesterone supplementation

Supplements for Insomnia
- Calcium and/or Magnesium, Zinc, Chromium and/or Gymnema
- Natural progesterone/estrogen supplementation
- Vitamin B complex
- Essential oils
- Valerian Root or Hops
- Liver detoxification program

Supplements for Digestive Problems
- Digestive enzymes and/or Hydrochloric acid (HCl)
- Probiotics and/or fiber
- Essential oils (Omega-3)
- Liver detoxification program

Supplements for Low Libido
- Natural progesterone supplementation
- Flaxseeds or flaxseed oil and adrenal support

Supplements for Migraines
- Natural progesterone supplementation
- Ginkgo or Vitamin E complex (to thin the blood)
- Vitamin B complex (if caused by stress or low blood sugar)
- Essential oils (Omega-3)
- Magnesium (for relaxation)
- Liver detoxification program

Supplements for Hormonal Weight Gain
- Natural progesterone supplementation
- Chromium, Magnesium and Zinc
- Vitamin B complex (if caused by stress or low blood sugar)
- Essential oils (Omega-3)
- Thyroid and adrenal support
- Liver detoxification program

Supplements for Hair Loss
- Supplemental protein
- Natural progesterone supplementation
- Multiple mineral support
- Vitamin B complex (if caused by stress or low blood sugar)
- Essential oils (Omega-3)
- Thyroid and adrenal support
- Liver detoxification program

Supplements for Stress
- Antioxidants (Vitamins A, C, E and selenium)
- Magnesium
- Vitamin B complex
- Essential oils (Omega-3 fats)
- Eleuthero Root (Siberian Ginseng by Medi-Herb)
- Panax Ginseng and/or Licorice Root
- Withania (Ashwaganda by Medi-Herb)
- Gymnema and/or Chromium GTF

Be encouraged that making the suggested changes in this book can and will help you regain your hormonal balance.

May God bless you on your journey to hormonal health!

Endnotes

1. Sherrill Sellman, *Hormone Heresy* (Tulsa, OK: GetWell International, 2000), pp. 31-42.

2. Dr. Janet Lang, The New Balancing Female Hormones Seminar, 2003, pp. 135-137.

3. John Lee, M.D., *What Your Doctor May Not Tell You About Menopause* (New York, NY: Warner Books, 1996), p. 28.

4. Sherrill Sellman, pp. 4-5.

5. John Lee, M.D., *What Your Doctor May Not Tell You About Premenopause* (New York, NY: Warner Books, 1999), pp. 99-101.

6. Shari Lieberman, *Get Off the Menopause Roller Coaster* (New York, NY: Avery, 2000), p. 24.

7. Dr. Janet Lang, The New Balancing Female Hormones Seminar, 2003, p. 13.

8. Lee, pp. 86-88.

9. Earl Mindell, Ph.D., *Prescription Alternatives* (Los Angeles, CA: Keats Publishing, 1998), pp. 21-22.

10. Nancy Beckham, "Why Women Should Not Take HRT," *WellBeing Magazine,* No. 67, p. 70.

11. *John Lee Medical Letter*, July 2002, p. 3.

12. Gorman, Christina and Park, Alice, "The Truth About Hormones," *Time Magazine*, July 22, 2002, cover story, pp. 33-36.

13. Dr. Johnathan Wright, *Natural Hormone Replacement* (Petaluma, CA: Smart Publications, 1997), p. 23.

14. Liz Grist, Ph.D., *A Woman's Guide to Alternative Medicine* (Chicago, IL: Contemporary Books, Inc., 1988), pp. 52, 53, 56.

15. Dr. Janet Lang, The New Balancing Female Hormones Seminar, 2003, p. 39.

16. Gary Null, *Women's Health Solutions* (New York, NY: Seven Stories Press, 2002), p. 490.

17. Ibid. p. 490.

18. Sellman, p. 72.

19. Null, p. 490.

20. Sellman, pp. 78-79.

21. Null, p. 102.

22. *Taber's Cyclopedic Medical Dictionary,* 1997.

23. Sellman, p. 17.

24. Sellman, pp. 43-47.

25. John Lee, M.D., *What Your Doctor May Not Tell You About Menopause* (New York, NY: Warner Books, 1996), p. 189.

26. Dr. Susan Love, *Dr. Susan Love's Hormone Book* (New York, NY: Three River's Press, 1997), p. 127.

27. Love, p. 109.

28. *Journal of the American Medical Association (JAMA),* 2003, 289:2651-2662.

29. Carl Germano, *The Osteoporosis Solution* (New York, NY: Kensington Books, 1999), p. 11.

30. Ibid, p. 11.

31. Love, p. 74.

32. Dr. Christiane Northrup, *The Wisdom of Menopause* (New York, NY: Bantam Books, 2001), pp. 377-380.

33. Lee, p. 152.

34. Lee, pp. 151-152.

35. Sellman, *Hormone Heresy Supplement*, p. 26.

36. Ibid.

37. Sandra Coney, *The Menopause Industry* (Victoria, Australia: Spinifex, 1993), p. 164.

38. Leslie Kenton, *Passage to Power* (London: Random House, 1995), pp. 19-20.

39. Sellman, *Hormone Heresy,* p. 26.

40. Ibid.

41. Mindell, p. 493.

42. Dr. John Lee Natural Hormone Balance Seminar Tapes.

43. John Lee, M.D., *What Your Doctor May Not Tell You About Breast Cancer* (New York, NY: Warner Books, 2002), p. 154.

44. Lee, pp. 160-161.

45. Linda Ojeda, Ph.D., *Menopause Without Medicine* (Alameda, CA: Hunter House, 1989), p. 37.

46. *John Lee Medical Letter*, July 2001.

47. Jonn Matsen, N. D., *The Mysterious Cause of Illness* (Canfield, OH: Fischer Publishing, 1987), pp. 7-9.

48. *Digestive Disease Weekly,* San Francisco, CA, May 23, 2002.

49. Dr. Larrian Gillespie, *The Menopause Diet* (Beverly Hills, CA: Healthy Life Publications, 1999), p.110.

50. John Lee, M.D., *What Your Doctor May Not Tell You About Premenopause* (New York, NY: Warner Books, 1999), p. 153-155.

51. Dr. Sandra Cabot, *The Healthy Liver and Bowel Book* (Cobbitty, Australia, 1999), pp. 17-18.

52. R. D. Gambrell, *Fertility and Sterility*, 1982: 37:457-74.

53. Raquel Martin, *The Estrogen Alternative* (Rochester, Vermont: Healing Arts Press, 1997), p. 47.

54. John Lee, M.D., *What Your Doctor May Not Tell You About Menopause* (New York, NY: Warner Books, 1996), p. 65.

55. Lee, pp. 62-64.

56. Dr. Bob Arnot, *The Breast Cancer Prevention Diet* (New York, NY: Little Brown and Co., 1998), p.67.

57. Sherrill Sellman, *Hormone Heresy Supplement,* pp. 18-25.

58. Arnot, p. 132.

59. Arnot, p. 98.

60. Arnot, p. 53.

61. Arnot, p. 103.

62. John Lee, M.D., *What Your Doctor May Not Tell You About Premenopause* (New York, NY: Warner Books, 1999), p. 90.

63. John Lee, M.D,. *What Your Doctor May Not Tell You About Breast Cancer* (New York: Warner Books, 2002), p. 307.

64. Arnot, p. 103.

65. Sellman, p. 211.

66. John Lee, M.D., *What Your Doctor May Not Tell You About Premenopause* (New York, NY: Warner Books, 1999), p. 78.

67. Ibid, p. 275.

68. Arnot, p. 76.

69. John Lee, M.D., *What Your Doctor May Not Tell You About Menopause* (New York, NY: Warner Books, 1996), p. 281.

70. Arnot, p. 73.

71. Ibid.

72. Ibid.

I have made every effort possible to check the accuracy of material quoted. If there is any question, or a possible mistake in quoting of any material, necessary changes will be made in future editions.

Index

Order Form

Please Print

Name _____

Address _____

City _____ State _____ Zip _____

Phone _____

E-mail _____

METHOD OF PAYMENT

Check _____ Credit Card: Visa_____ Mastercard_____

Card number _____ Exp. date_____

Authorization Signature _____

ITEM	QTY	PRICE
Why Can't I Lose Weight? ($17.95)		
Why Can't I Lose Weight Cookbook ($17.95)		
Why Can't I Stay Motivated? ($14.95)		
Why Am I So Grumpy, Dopey and Sleepy? ($11.95)		
Why Am I So Wacky? ($11.95)		
Why Eat Like Jesus Ate? ($11.95)		
Why Do I Need Whole Food Supplements? ($9.95)		
Why Do I Feel So Lousy? ($9.95)		
Subtotal		
Shipping & Handling Add 15%		
(Add 8% if resident of OK) Tax		
Total		

Send check or money order to:

Life Design Nutrition

Lorrie Medford, CN

PO Box 54007

Tulsa, OK 74155

918-664-4483

918-664-0300 (fax)

E-mail orders: lorrie@lifedesignnutrition.com

www.lifedesignnutrition.com